chill out
& get
healthy

AIMEE E. RAUPP, M.S., L.Ac.

chill out
& get
healthy

live clean to
be **strong**
and stay *sexy*

 NEW AMERICAN LIBRARY

New American Library
Published by New American Library, a division of
Penguin Group (USA) Inc., 375 Hudson Street,
New York, New York 10014, USA
Penguin Group (Canada), 90 Eglinton Avenue East, Suite 700, Toronto, Ontario M4P 2Y3, Canada (a division of Pearson Penguin Canada Inc.) • Penguin Books Ltd., 80 Strand, London WC2R 0RL, England • Penguin Ireland, 25 St. Stephen's Green, Dublin 2, Ireland (a division of Penguin Books Ltd.) • Penguin Group (Australia), 250 Camberwell Road, Camberwell, Victoria 3124, Australia (a division of Pearson Australia Group Pty. Ltd.) • Penguin Books India Pvt. Ltd., 11 Community Centre, Panchsheel Park, New Delhi - 110 017, India • Penguin Group (NZ), 67 Apollo Drive, Rosedale, North Shore 0632, New Zealand (a division of Pearson New Zealand Ltd.) • Penguin Books (South Africa) (Pty.) Ltd., 24 Sturdee Avenue, Rosebank, Johannesburg 2196, South Africa

Penguin Books Ltd., Registered Offices:
80 Strand, London WC2R 0RL, England

First published by New American Library,
a division of Penguin Group (USA) Inc.

First Printing, August 2009
10 9 8 7 6 5 4 3 2 1

 REGISTERED TRADEMARK—MARCA REGISTRADA

LIBRARY OF CONGRESS CATALOGING-IN-PUBLICATION DATA:

Raupp, Aimee E.
 Chill out and get healthy: live clean to be strong and stay sexy/Aimee E. Raupp.
  p. cm.
 ISBN 978-0-451-22636-5
 1. Women—Health and hygiene—Popular works. I. Title.
 RA 778.R29 2009
 613'.04244—dc22   2009001699

Set in Joanna
Designed by Pauline Neuwirth

Printed in the United States of America

PUBLISHER'S NOTE
Every effort has been made to ensure that the information contained in this book is complete and accurate. However, neither the publisher nor the author is engaged in rendering professional advice or services to the individual reader. The ideas, procedures, and suggestions contained in this book are not intended as a substitute for consulting with your physician. All matters regarding your health require medical supervision. Neither the author nor the publisher shall be liable or responsible for any loss or damage allegedly arising from any information or suggestion in this book. The opinions expressed in this book represent the personal views of the author and not of the publisher.
 The recipes contained in this book are to be followed exactly as written. The publisher is not responsible for your specific health or allergy needs that may require medical supervision. The publisher is not responsible for any adverse reactions to the recipes contained in this book.
 The publisher does not have any control over and does not assume any responsibility for author or third-party Web sites or their content.

To Mom, Dad and three hundred months

acknowledgments

$\mathcal{I}$ AM BEYOND grateful to Harry, Lili and Sam, who continue to shower me with undying love and support. I love you. Thank you.

A special thanks to Kimmy, Danielle, Siobhan, Johanna, Melanie, Jessica, Hima, Nathalie, Ali, Kymber, Brooke, Athena, Sasha, Penny, Marilyn, Monroe, Aunt Eileen, Auntie and Uncle Ed for your constant feedback, love, laughter, patience and encouragement.

To Sloane Miller, I couldn't have done this without you. I am forever indebted to your genius.

To Michelle Wolfson for believing in this project from the get-go, for making it happen and for holding my hand along the way.

To Tracy Bernstein and everyone at NAL and Penguin Group for taking on this project with such enthusiasm and pride.

To Piper Weiss for your gentle yet profound guidance. I love you.

To Megan Driscoll for helping bring my dreams to life.

To Naomi Lewis for your tremendous generosity, knowledge and friendship.

Thank you to my patients, teachers and mentors for perpetually inspiring me to find the way.

Thank you to the events in my life—both good and bad—that filled me with the passion and desire to do whatever I can do to make this world a better place.

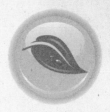

contents

HOW TO USE THIS BOOK

*L*ADIES, IT'S TIME to Chill Out and Get Healthy. It's time to get your health into kick-ass shape.

Are you that crazed, irritable, cry-at-the-drop-of-a-hat, raging-PMS girl?

Do you have that I'm-so-bloated-it's-uncomfortable tummy after every meal?

Are you scared that you're not going to be fertile when it's time to get preggers?

Are you exhausted every morning and absolutely *need* that double no-foam latte to wake your ass up?

Do you have that I-haven't-taken-a-poop-in-three-days consti-pated feeling every single day?

Are you taking an antidepressant? An antianxiety med? A pill to help you sleep? A pill to help you poop? All of the above?

Are you so stressed-out that you feel like you have no time to get to the grocery store, pick up your dry cleaning or make that overdue phone call to your mother?

Do you think soy is good for you and eat it in every form: tofu, soy milk, SoyJoy bars?

Are you a regular at Sephora because every time you look in the mirror, you think you see another wrinkle?

If you answered yes to any one of those questions, *Chill Out & Get Healthy* was written for YOU. I know you really want to, *need* to, maintain your sanity, live healthfully, age gracefully and prevent disease amid the chaos of today's world, and this book will show you how.

Chill Out & Get Healthy is a fabulous-new-you lifestyle guide—and not a jump-on-the-bandwagon two-week diet fad—that will teach you how to nourish both your body and soul, decrease general anxiety, manage overwhelming stressors, maintain and improve your fertility, beautify your skin from the inside out, get your digestive system back on track and fight the fear of oh-my-God-is-that-another-wrinkle aging.

By giving you practical, modern-day twists on ancient Chinese Medicine theories and traditions, this antiaging, anti-getting-sickly-and-crotchety lifestyle guide will empower you with the knowledge and tools to manage your health today and avoid the unfortunate and all-too-common tumultuous, drug-dependent path of I'm-not-feeling-so-hot health.

And it will help you do all this RIGHT NOW!

So dig in and read this book from beginning to end. Read it in the order in which it was written, as the information presented builds upon itself.

Go on, girl, get your read on and get on the Chill Out and Get Healthy train. Start putting to use all the easy-to-follow advice, age-old and avant-garde tips and inspirational you-can-do-it cajoling right NOW. This book is the how-to guide to your health. It will show you how your lifestyle—what you eat, how you manage your stress, how much you sleep, how often you poop, how you dealt with your last heartbreak—directly, totally, one hundred percent, without a doubt affects your physical and mental health.

Read this book, get your health in gear, maintain your hotness, battle wrinkles and gray hairs, have a daily bowel movement that leaves you feeling oh-so-good and change your life NOW. Get on board with the Chill Out and Get Healthy lifestyle or you risk becoming an irritable, pill-popping, wrinkled, overweight, constipated and unhappy lady, and that definitely isn't sexy!

Keep in mind, the information in this book is NOT a substitute for medical care and shouldn't be used as such. I encourage you to work with a team of health-care providers, alternative and mainstream, Eastern and Western. I want you to find your best solutions for whatever ails you. I invite you to be in charge of your health. If at any point you have questions, go to my Web site, www. aimeeraupp.com, e-mail me or check out my biweekly blog for information on common health-care issues.

Ladies, I am calling on you to Chill Out and Get Healthy NOW! So go on, sink your teeth into this book and get your health into rock-solid shape!

who's this girl?

I'M AIMEE RAUPP, the author of this book. I became obsessed with educating my fabulously feminine peers about chilling out and getting healthy NOW one Sunday at brunch with my girlfriends. I remember looking around the table at my girls, who on the surface all looked so great, so beautiful and so New York City chic: friend "A" with her new blond highlights, Invisaligned teeth and toned biceps, friend "B" with her newest plush pink lip gloss and her hot Theory jeans and friend "C" with her dark black locks, her beautiful complexion and those sexy new boots she purchased on a recent trip to London.

But here's the thing: despite their seeming perfection, I knew that deep down their health was suffering. As beautiful and unruffled as friend A is, she constantly battles an acidic stomach, tension headaches and bouts of insomnia; friend B gets chronic yeast infections and has quasi-allergic reactions to *some* of her boyfriends during sex; and friend C spends a chunk of her day rushing to the bathroom to relieve her cramped and bloated tummy.

Like you, they are all smart enough to realize that their health needs help. Like you, they are looking for answers beyond "Take this or that pill." When we talked about their health that Sunday afternoon, I told them, just as I am telling you now, "Listen, if you are sick now or suffering with minor ailments, you're probably in poor health. Not to stress you out even more, but seriously, you have got to get a grip on your health NOW before you turn into a wrinkled and bloated old lady who depends on ten medications a day to get by. Come on, ladies, you can do it!"

Do you want to be healthy and hot at fifty? Or do you want to be that wrinkled and bloated old lady at fifty? The choice is yours to make.

I'm assuming since you picked up this book, you'd like to maintain your hotness and your health. I'd like to help you.

As an experienced practitioner of Traditional Chinese Medicine, both professionally and personally, I have valuable and practical advice on health to give you. I use acupuncture, herbs, diet and lifestyle modifications to ward off the scary, creepy, crawly, crotchety things that haunt my patients.

Chinese Medicine (CM) is about helping people live a more comfortable, more content, more harmonious life, not just externally, but internally. It teaches people how to get their health and their life back into balance, not just for today, but for the long haul.

What I do for a living is make people healthier and help prevent disease. I do this by sticking little hair-thin needles into specific acupuncture points on the body to release Qi (an imperative substance in our bodies that allows us to function properly, pronounced Chee), educating people about the importance of their health, diet and lifestyle choices, and prescribing herbs to assist body function.

I can already hear you: "Don't the needles hurt?" or "Is this some kind of cult?" or my all-time favorite, "Isn't that voodoo?" The answer is no, no AND no! Just because I use needles and practice an ancient Eastern science doesn't mean I walk around in a yellow robe chanting, nor does it mean that I'll make you chant (although I may offer you a mantra or two). I chose this profession because preventing disease speaks to me. Or, put another way, I pursued a higher education in Traditional Chinese Medicine because the idea of death and aging scares the shit out of me, like it does most of us. I will do everything in my power to avoid becoming that sick and cantankerous old lady taking ten medications! I'm here to help you do the same.

In order for me to be good, really good, at my job, I need to speak, eat, live and breathe my medicine; by doing so, I have learned how to balance my health and my life. I practice what I preach while managing my finances, a practice in New York City, a second practice in Nyack, New York, and a busy girl's social calendar, training for half-marathons and triathlons, writing books, eating healthy, meditating and staying sane.

I believe in making the best choices possible and I believe that choosing health over disease is the only choice we can make.

I didn't always think this way. Once upon a time, I was where you are now. I was crazed, irritable, feeling unfocused and dragging my feet on a daily basis. I had lifeless hair, dry skin and puffy dark circles under my eyes that no one-hundred-dollar vitamin-K-enriched eye cream from Sephora could fix. But I recovered and I'm telling you, you can too. You can manage your life and be healthy. It's not that hard. I am also telling you that no one is perfect, and that I still struggle with living healthy, but about eighty to eighty-five percent of the time, I succeed at it. And that's enough time to get the job done.

When I was first introduced to Chinese Medicine, I was twenty-five, and I was far—really far—from "health." I was studying neuroscience at the San Diego campus of the University of California (UCSD). I had graduated from Rutgers University with a degree in biology and my hopes were to be a medical doctor. As I made my way into the field, it began to make its way out of me. I sat day in and day out in a windowless room, growing cells in a petri dish, researching the causes of Alzheimer's disease. Was amyloid beta-protein the cause of Alzheimer's disease? My profound theory was, "Well, maybe." My own grandmother was in a nursing home, suffering inhumanly with Alzheimer's; I wanted to save her life and I couldn't. The fact that what I was doing wouldn't immediately affect her life killed me.

At that point in time, my life consisted of working like a dog, a fairly temperamental relationship with my live-in boyfriend, somewhat serious bouts of depression and the daily struggle of an eating disorder. On top of it, I had eczema everywhere, I was constantly bloated, my energy sucked and alcohol and running were my only solaces.

I was questioning my future and myself. I was despondent, yet I really had no idea of it. My depression was sitting there screaming at me and I just wasn't listening. Like most of us, I held a deaf ear to my emotions, to my insides, to what my body was telling me.

Finally, I sought out CM because I wanted relief from my chronic eczema that seemed to be spreading to every corner of my body. Chinese Medicine's macroscopic approach to health gave me hope because unfortunately Western medicine's microscopic antics were failing me. It was during that first acupuncture session that I realized how much everyday suffering I was personally experiencing. I didn't have just chronic eczema. I was really, really far from health. I realized that I had to fix myself before I could ever doctor anyone else.

At my first acupuncture session I was a cocky twenty-five-year-old neurobiology grad student and research scientist who was eager for help, yet skeptical of this "foreign" medicine. I remember the acupuncturist asking what I had eaten for breakfast. "A Balance Bar," I boasted, thinking that was a great and healthful choice. I was also secretly proud of myself for not vomiting that morning, as I was still struggling with bulimia.

"That's not food," she said, disappointingly.

In CM, the number one place Qi comes from is the food we ingest and the air we breathe in. In fact, the Chinese symbol for Qi depicts the steam that rises above rice as you cook it. We need to eat alive and fresh foods so that we can generate the healthiest of Qi, and we definitely shouldn't be puking our food up!

Then the acupuncturist felt my pulses and said, "Your blood is VERY deficient."

How could she tell? I wondered. I remember at one point being told I was anemic, but how did she know? All she was doing was feeling my pulse and looking at my tongue, my eyes and my skin.

"Are you a vegetarian?"

"Yes!"

"That explains why your blood is so weak. … Do you ever crave meat or protein?"

"Umm … I guess?"

Honestly, I craved meat often. But thinking I was doing the right thing by being a vegetarian, I ignored those cravings. Often I would snack on peanut butter (processed, store-bought and definitely not organic) to satisfy the meat craving. Sometimes I would actually dream about eating a hamburger!

"Why are you a vegetarian?"

"Because I thought it was healthy to be a vegetarian." Secretly, I didn't eat meat because I thought it was fattening.

She then pushed around on my stomach, asking if certain areas were tender.

"When was your last bowel movement?"

"Yesterday, I think?"

"Normal bowel movements should occur one to three times per day, be well formed and easy to pass and leave you feeling completely voided. What are your bowel movements like?"

Suddenly I had a flashback to yesterday's study session at Starbucks. I was drinking my usual: a Grande coffee with raspberry syrup and a fair amount of (nonorganic, hormone-filled) milk. About ten minutes after I finished my first of two coffees, I had to immediately make my way to the bathroom to take a very urgent and explosive poop.

"I think my bowels are a bit irregular," I said.

After my first acupuncture treatment, she gave me homework for the week: I was to ask my body if it wanted meat and then meditate on the answer.

Meditate, I wondered. Who has time for meditation?

With her well-informed direction and kind patience, I ultimately did as I was told: I learned how to meditate; I started eating meat; I asked my body what it needed and began treating myself better—I made everyday lifestyle choices that led me in the direction of better health. With her guidance, I began to take control of my health and heal myself. The end result was earth-shattering: my eczema improved and was under my control, I became a ravenous carnivore who eventually got a handle on her bulimia, I dropped my studies at UCSD, I broke off my relationship and I pursued higher education in Traditional Chinese Medicine.

Almost a decade later, I am the acupuncturist. Day in and day out I direct patients to meditate, to eat better, to live healthfully, to take life in stride and to reprioritize. Day in and day out, I encourage them to take care and choose health NOW. Day in and day out I empower them with the tools to age gracefully and live disease free.

Let me explain what I mean by disease because it's probably a bit different from how you're used to thinking about it. In Western society, having a disease means having a medical condition like cancer or emphysema. However, in CM we define disease by breaking down the word:

"dis" = the absence of something
"ease" = peace, harmony, comfort, contentment, enjoyment, tranquility

Simply put, "dis-ease" is defined by the absence of harmony. Diseases range from minor physical symptoms to major ones, from quirky little emotional outbursts to the big ol' emotional pain that we so brilliantly suppress.

Here are some examples of CM dis-eases:

Anxiety, depression, PMS, menstrual cramping, constipation, diarrhea, night sweats, jaw grinding (TMJ), headaches, pain (as in back pain, neck pain, knee pain), fatigue, the inability to concentrate, panic attacks, insomnia, palpitations, bloating and gas.

In CM any "dis-ease" experienced on a fairly consistent basis is a sign of a body in not-so-great health.

So tell me, how many of those symptoms do you experience in any given week? Then tell me how healthy you think you are.

Listen, don't you ever wonder what all these symptoms mean? It must mean *something* when every morning you wake up with a headache, or with a feeling of complete exhaustion. It must mean *something* when you have such bad anxiety that you can't get on an elevator. Or tell me this, did you ever wonder why it is that you need a cup of coffee each day to have a bowel movement?

Tell me about the state of your bowels, the quality of your sleep, your ability to manage your stress levels, or the viability of the food you ate today.

Tell me honestly, how healthy do you think you are?

With this book, I will teach you how to slow down and feel your health, your happiness, your sadness and your anxiety. This book will teach you how to recognize that your emotions, lifestyle, diet and health are not separate entities. They are all interdependent, and you are in fact one unit.

For the most part we recognize that our poor diets will have physical manifestations (i.e., we will gain weight, get cellulite or break out). We need to realize that our broken hearts will also have physical manifestations. We need to acknowledge that our stressful jobs will have physical manifestations. That our poor sleep will have physical manifestations. We need to slow down enough to take inventory of our insides and understand why it is we are broken. We need to take a deep breath once in a while and assess how we really feel on the inside. We need to taste our food and identify whether it is giving us indigestion. We need to pay attention while we are driving, noticing how much tension we may be holding in our neck and arms as we grip the steering wheel. Seriously. We need to relax, restore and take the time to regain control of our health!

"No freaking way," you say. "I don't have any extra time."

Well, to that I say, **You better make time for it.** Don't worry, doll—I'll show you how, because you need to get back in touch with yourself. Your health is at stake.

You have to start living knowing that life with poor health is the pits and it's only gonna get worse!

You need to begin treating your body, your precious, only-one-life-to-live body, like the palace that it is.

I can promise you good, even great health, now and in the future, if you just invest a little time and energy into it on a daily basis, start-ing NOW.

In the pages that follow, I will teach you simple everyday choices that you can and should make for yourself; simple everyday choices that will help you optimize your health and make your life, right here, right now, dramatically better.

I'll teach you how to make the healthy, responsible, oh-I-feel-so-good choice (and how to actually feel good about it). Like, green tea or your double nonfat, no-foam soy latte? Ambien or a nighttime meditation? Zoloft and Xanax or therapy? Processed or organic? Mi-crowaved or slow-cooked? Get it?

I'll also teach you how to chill out every day, not just when you're on a beach somewhere or when you have a cocktail in your hand (I call it Chill the F**k Out time—you'll learn all about it in chapter 3).

There are three things that you are going to hear me say over and over and over again, until I'm blue in the face and until I feel that you have heard me. These three things are the key to true health. They are the best antiaging tools you'll ever come across; they are imperative in keeping you strong, healthy and sexy.

1. Eat clean, organic and nondead foods.
2. Sleep seven to eight hours a night. Period.
3. Chill the F**k Out for at least five minutes each day.

Not so hard, right?

OK, ladies, one last thing before you read on: I do not have a magic wand, nor does anyone else (and if people say they do, they are lying). All I have is knowledge to share and the desire to em-power you to change your health. But FYI: this will take work. This is a process. You cannot sit on your couch watching lame-ass reality TV and expect me to change your health for you. That, my dear, is your job. I am just here to hold your hand (and maybe scream at you once in a while, but I promise, it's all outta love!).

Well then, let's get on with it. Let's get on that hot and healthy, antiaging, staying-sexy-and-sane train!

2.

DO YOU KNOW
what Healthy is?

$\mathcal{L}$ADIES, HERE'S THE philosophy to live by:

**A body in great health is like that gorgeous Marc Jacobs bag
featured in *In Style* last month—durable, dependable,
functional, always looking and feeling oh-so-fabulous
and envied by all.**

Joanna, a thirty-three-year-old television producer, came in carrying a beautiful, oversized Cole Haan basket-weave brown leather tote. As she put down her handbag filled with God knows what, she told me how she was suffering with neck and shoulder tension. Funny how she made no connection between her pain and the huge boulder strapped to her shoulder. As I asked her all sorts of questions, she sighed and rolled her eyes; basically, she thought my questions were completely unrelated to her pain. *Au contraire!* I asked about her medical history, what she ate for breakfast, the frequency and consistency of her bowel movements and the quality of her sleep. Based on the dark circles under her eyes, the way she constantly sighed when she spoke and the ruddiness of her skin, I knew there was more going on with her internal and external health than she was aware of. That's the beauty of CM: seemingly inconsequential details actually reveal a great deal of information regarding the condition of one's overall health.

In CM, the ambiguous symptoms you live with on a daily basis, like the inability to sleep or pooping only twice a week, add up to a bigger picture and give practitioners like me an overall impression of the state of your health. The principles of CM view an individual's health along a macroscopic spectrum, rather than by microscopic laboratory results. You remember "macro" from your college econ class: "macro" is the large system, the overall, the total structure; "micro" is the tiniest part, the infinitesimal details. My job is to ask you a lot of questions in order to piece together all your symptoms and random complaints so that I can understand why your body isn't working properly. It's basically nosy detective work: I sniff and search and look under every surface so that I can help you bring your health and YOU back to the fabulous place they long to be.

After I spoke with Joanna, it was clear that her ruddy complexion was the result of her constipated digestive system. Man, the poor girl rarely poops! The dark circles under her eyes are because she sleeps only five hours each night, even when she takes an Ambien. Her constant sighing has to do with the fact that she is tense and irritable because she hates her job. It's no wonder she's in pain—besides carrying around an oversized handbag and being sleep deprived, she's carrying the weight of her world in her neck and shoulders.

Any of this sound familiar?

Here are some nosy-detective-esque questions for you to answer so that we can get you back to fabulous health—inside and out!

Do you wake up in the morning feeling refreshed?
Do you have at least one well-formed and easy-to-pass bowel
    movement each day?

Do you have enough energy to get through the day (without the need for caffeine or sugar)?

Do you wake up hungry in the morning?

Can you fall asleep and stay asleep without the need for medication or alcohol?

Do you remember the last time you didn't get irrational and irritable before your period?

Can you make it through a day without feeling gassy or bloated?

If you answered, "No way, Aimee!" to any *one* of these questions, your body isn't nearly as fabulous and healthy as you think it is.

Don't feel bad. Unfortunately, very few of us know how a healthy body should feel. Has anyone ever sat down with you and told you that it's not normal to be foggy-headed in the morning or bloated after a meal on a consistent basis? We all know that we are supposed to sleep between seven and eight hours per night (even though we don't) and that we really shouldn't suffer with aches and pains even on a nongym day (even though we do). But what about the other stuff? Has anyone ever told you what your bowel movements should look like, before Dr. Oz on *Oprah* did? Or that horrendous, I'm-embarrassed-to-leave-my-house gas is not normal? Has anyone ever told you that this whole PMS thing is manageable and dare I say avoidable? Or that a normally functioning body should have enough energy to get through the day without that afternoon trip to Dunkin' Donuts?

In this chapter I am going to walk you through what true health should look and feel like. This chapter is kind of like your own personal health road map. It's going to take you on a little guided tour of your body and your health so that you can pinpoint the areas that are out of whack and in need of a fixin'. Some of the information here is obvious—and is by no means meant to be demeaning to you or your knowledge of health. I'm just laying down some groundwork. The rest of the chapters in this book will give you all sorts of realistic ancient Chinese not-so-secret tips you can start applying today to get your body back to that state of oh-so-freakin'-fabulous health!

• SLEEPING BEAUTY HAD IT RIGHT •

You should be getting seven or eight hours of sleep every night.

I'm going to say it again, because it's that important:

You need seven or eight hours of sleep every night!

NO SLEEP = OBESITY AND DEATH

Chronic sleep deprivation is a leading cause of any and all diseases in our society. In laboratory studies, rats who aren't allowed to sleep begin dying after five days. Seriously. Scientists at the University of Chicago Pritzker School of Medicine found that within six days people who slept only four hours a night were unable to regulate their blood sugar levels, predisposing them to type 2 diabetes! These subjects were also really, really hungry, so hungry that the scientists hypothesized that sleep deprivation is a cause of the American obesity epidemic! Research scientists at the University of Pennsylvania and Texas Tech University have found links between short sleep times and obesity, heart disease, high blood pressure and stroke. Researchers at Harvard concluded that women who sleep less than six hours each night are more susceptible to cancer and cardiovascular disease, have weaker immune systems and have an overall increased chance of dying in comparison to their peers who sleep seven to eight hours each night. Darlin', you need to get seven to eight hours of shut-eye!

SPIRIT IN THE NIGHT

Not only does sleeping keep us alive and disease free; it keeps us sane. In CM, we see sleep as being not just physically restorative but emotionally imperative as well. When we are asleep, our body rests but so does our spirit, which in CM theory is the "treasure that gives brightness to life and is responsible for consciousness and mental abilities." Without ample sleep, your spirit can't rest. And since your spirit brings brightness to your life and is responsible for consciousness and mental abilities … when your spirit is tired and sleep deprived, you will become a crazy and anxious person with no mental vitality and a dull life!

Western medical research supports this CM notion; sleep-deprived individuals display a disconnection between the emotional region of the brain and the region of the brain that controls rational thought and decision making. So according to both Western medicine and CM, sleep deprivation makes you a moody, illogical, emotional and overreactive lunatic. Girl, get to sleep, already!

WAH-WAH

"But I don't have time to sleep eight hours!" I hear you moan.

Make time! You need sleep! It is really the only time that the body gets to restore itself.

You should not need to take medication to sleep. You should not regularly have wild, vivid dreams that you remember or jaw-clenching nightmares that make your heart race. You should not wake up with a headache or a chipped tooth from grinding your teeth all night. You should more often than not awake in the morning feeling refreshed and ready to start your day. You should not have bags under your eyes from sleep deprivation.

Chapter 9 has some great, simple tips on improving your sleep!

• HUNGRY LIKE THE WOLF •

HONOR YOUR HUNGER

Bottom line: you should get hungry and you should eat. Period.

Hunger arises when your glycogen (the body's primary short-term energy source) falls below its threshold, stimulating the brain to tell you to eat. The sensation of hunger, in a normally functioning body, should come on a couple of hours after your last meal. The way you satisfy this sensation is to eat. It's not rocket science. Eating every couple of hours is what your body wants to do. It's what it needs to do. Ladies, you must honor your hunger.

When you are honoring your hunger, you should wake up and want to eat breakfast (or get hungry directly after you have your first, no-need-for-coffee, well-formed, easy-to-pass poop of the day).

EAT BREAKFAST

Scientists at the University of Minnesota found that adolescents who eat breakfast have a lower body mass index than those who don't. So, sweetie, don't skip breakfast or you'll gain weight. I'm not joking. Eating a healthful breakfast stimulates your metabolism and keeps it going like a stallion of a workhorse throughout the day.

THEN, EAT AGAIN

After eating breakfast, your body should get hungry every couple of hours. This tells us that your body has an efficient metabolism. A body that is starved all day long has zilch for a metabolism and over time will gain weight and hold on to it. Eat!

NEVER IGNORE YOUR HUNGER

You cannot ignore your hunger, because when you don't eat, your body loses its primary source of energy: food. Without energy, metabolic rate becomes embarrassingly slow, you lose the ability to absorb nutrition from your food (if and when you decide to eat), your body holds on to excess weight and your vital organs begin to shrink! Seriously, starvation is disgusting and it leads to total-body shutdown, weight gain because your metabolic rate slows to an almost complete stop and eventually DEATH. No joke.

One more thing: if you are struggling with an eating disorder where you don't want to eat (or you are puking up your food) for fear of weight gain or you are habitually overeating, YOU MUST GET PROFESSIONAL HELP. Believe me, I was there once. Eating disorders are horrible and they should not have a place in your life anymore. They are life suckers and they age the crap out of you.

QUENCH YOUR THIRST

You should be thirsty, not only after a night of drinking, but on a daily basis. You should be able to quench your thirst. Your primary fluid intake should be water, and approximately half your body weight in ounces of water; for example, if your weight is 130 pounds, you should be taking in 65 ounces of water a day! (If you have only one kidney, drink just one-fourth your weight in ounces.)

Water should, for the most part, be drunk at room temperature, as, according to CM theory, water that is too cold will slow down your metabolism.

Huh?

Yes, cold water will slow down your metabolism. Did you ever experience a tummyache after drinking a cold glass of water? This is because your internal temperature is approximately 98.6 degrees Fahrenheit and cold water from the fridge is about 35 degrees Fahrenheit. When something that is more than 60 degrees colder than your internal temperature enters your system, it shocks the system, causing stomach cramping and a slow metabolism. Before your body can do anything else, it must first warm up this cold water. Only then can it get back to its job of maintaining your metabolism, getting the imperative nutrients it needs from the foods you eat and burning fat!

Drink room-temperature plain water. Stuff like Vitaminwater, Gatorade, coffee, Crystal Light and Diet Coke does NOT count as water. I don't even think they count as anything besides gross toxic sugary stuff! But, more on that in chapters 5 and 6.

SO SMOOTH

Digestion should be easy, comfortable and gas free. You should be able to eat something, feel satisfied and move on. You should not crave something sweet after each meal. If you do, chances are you're not eating enough protein. You should not have to belch, fart, unbutton your pants or take a Tums after eating. If you do, guess what: you're not properly digesting your food.

FOOD FOR THOUGHT

Here's something to ponder: CM theory preaches that one should only eat when eating; this means you shouldn't be walking down the street eating, or driving and eating, or working and eating. Just eat when you eat! I know this is the land of the ultimate multi-taskers, but try chilling out when you're eating. Not to get all hokey on you, but try being grateful for the food that is in front of you; try tasting your food, smelling it, enjoying it. When you take your time to eat, you allow your body the energy to digest your food.

TOOT, TOOT

Belching or farting is a clear-cut sign of indigestion. These lovely little bubbles are your body's odorific way of saying "Hey, lady, I can't metabolize this food!" If you are experiencing smelly toot-toots or foul burps on a regular basis, you are probably eating too many indigestible foods like soy and dairy (more on that in chapter 5). Either that or you are eating way too fast and doing other things while you're eating. Or maybe you're doing all of the above?

• • •

SO-SEXY BLOATED BELLY, NOT

Bloating is uncomfortable and obnoxious and it just shouldn't happen. Not to mention that the loud rumbles that accompany bloating can be awfully embarrassing. The so-sexy bloat is usually a sign that either you've eaten too much or you cannot digest whatever you've just eaten.

Bloating is one step further down the line of poor digestion from gas and typically the two go together. Prolonged inefficient digestion—as a result of months or years of eating indigestible gas-olicious substances—causes food to accumulate in your gut, along with liquid and gas; this slows down the metabolic process, rendering you uncomfortably bloated and gassy after each meal because your body is so backed up! Sometimes your poor backed-up tummy is still digesting food you ate last week! Ewww!

AND IT BURNS, BURNS, BURNS

Reflux is yet another step further along the spectrum of poor digestion, showing us that not only has food accumulated in the gut, but now the overflow of last week's food is causing the stomach acid to brim over into your esophagus; it's like your digestive tract is a bubbly cauldron filled with undigested food that's overflowing and spilling out of the pot. That spillage is acid reflux. Yum.

Bottom line: a healthy and free-flowing digestive system should not experience any sort of indigestion on a regular basis and especially not with each meal.

Read more about improving your digestion in chapters 5, 6 and 9.

• POOPING •

BROWN BANANAS ARE BEAUTIFUL

When you have an efficient digestive system with enough Qi, you poop on a daily basis—or at least five days per week—and you shouldn't need a cup of coffee to do it! Bowel movements should be formed in one six-inch-or-so-long banana-like piece; it should pass out of you smoothly without sweat, grunts or groans. It shouldn't be urgent or explosive. It should leave you feeling completely evacuated. It shouldn't be watery or mucusy or have visible undigested food particles in it (unless you've had yourself some corn). It shouldn't be hard, dry or in the form of little pebbles. It should be brown. Not green. Not yellow.

Ladies, did you know that a daily, banana-like, brown bowel movement represents a strapping immune system? Now you do.

TIMING

According to Chinese Medicine theory, our first bowel movement should occur between five and seven a.m. Some people have up to three bowel movements a day. But one healthy, solid, easy-to-pass and oh-so-good-feeling poop each day is a sign of great health.

TAKE A LOOK-SEE

Girlfriend, do yourself a favor: the next time you do number two—check out what it looks like. I'm sure you already know this, but your bowel movements say a lot about the state of your health.

FREE THE POOP

Taking laxatives, doing enemas or ingesting other medications to help you go number two are fine for the short term, meaning once—max twice—a year. If you are doing any one of these things to help you defecate more than twice annually, you're robbing your body of its normal pooping capability. Taking aggressive things like laxatives on a regular basis negatively affects your metabolism: you are not allowing your body to properly digest things on its own. Abusing laxatives could be a sign of an eating disorder, and believe me, eating disorders ain't pretty. If this is you, see someone; get help; kick the bad habit—it's ruining your health and you're aging the shit out of yourself, literally! Sweetie, when your metabolism is abused in such a way, it inherently slows down and you will gain weight and have a hard time losing it (not to mention the damage you're doing to your precious body by depriving it of the nutrients it needs). Don't depend on these types of things to go to the bathroom. They are Band-Aid treatments. Get to the root of the problem and poop on your own. Free the Poop! It's liberating!

MORONIC COLONICS

Getting regular colonics is moronic! This überintrusive experience may be helpful or beneficial on a very infrequent basis (say, once or twice a lifetime, not six times a year!). When done repeatedly, they can really harm the musculature of your colon. How? You remember the tried-and-true saying "Use it or lose it." The same applies to the muscles of your colon. If you are depending on a colonic to clean out your colon, you are not allowing the muscles of your colon to work on their own. And the more you use colonics or other colon-cleansing methods, the less capable your body is when it comes to moving your poop out on its own.

Again, read more about improving your digestion and your ability to go number two in chapters 5, 6 and 9.

• TINKLING •

Pee should be pale yellow to clear in color (unless you've been eating beets). It should not be neon yellow, dark yellow or any other color for that matter. It should not be cloudy or have a strong odor (unless, of course, you've been eating asparagus). It should be consistent with your fluid intake, meaning if you drink a lot of water, you will be peeing a lot. Pee should not be urgent. Nor in your twenties and thirties should it leak out of you when you laugh or wake you up in the middle of the night (unless you're pregnant or you drank a big glass of water right before bed).

Urinary tract infections (UTIs) and bladder infections should not be a *regular* part of your existence. After a weekend with loads of sex, sure, you can get an infection—but really, you shouldn't. If these perils are occurring too often, chances are your immune system is weak, you are eating way too much sugar and your digestion is inefficient—leaving your gut loaded with an overgrowth of unhealthy bacteria.

Learn how to ward off these infections in chapter 9.

· THAT TIME OF THE MONTH ·

Listen up, girls: we do NOT need to suffer when we have our period. We should not have debilitating cramps, or a depression so deep that it scares our mothers. We should not need medication to get through our period: not Advil or Motrin, not Xanax, not your antidepressant of choice. We should not crave chocolate so badly that we're willing to give up our big toe for some. And we should not bleed so heavily that we stain clothing, bleed through a super Tampax before leaving the house in the morning or pass clots so big that we feel like we're giving birth.

There shouldn't be spotting at any point outside of your monthly period.

When your period comes, you shouldn't get pimples, you shouldn't get diarrhea or constipation, you shouldn't get insomnia or night sweats, you shouldn't have extreme mood swings or headaches and you definitely shouldn't need to take the day off from work.

Seriously, this whole premenstrual syndrome complex does not need to be the bane of our existence. You can make changes in your life that will allay your monthly suffering. And NO, I am not referring to taking the birth control pill! Taking the Pill does not get to the root of the problem and can have other side effects (more on that in chapter 7). I am talking about lifestyle and dietary changes you can implement that will make you feel like a natural (and pain-free) woman!

According to the principles of CM, a healthy and balanced female does not have PMS.

"Whoa! What?" I hear you say.

PMS in Chinese Medicine is the result of stuck liver energy.

"A stuck liver? What the heck is that?"

The liver energy gets stuck when we eat too many toxic, indigestible substances (like processed foods, alcohol and prescription or recreational drugs). The liver also gets hampered and stagnant when we repress our emotions. Girlfriend, strike a pose and express yourself (learn how in chapter 4)!

Your periods should come regularly and be between twenty-eight and thirty-two days apart (where the first day of bleeding is day one of your cycle). They should come on quietly, with slight breast tenderness and very little cramping. They should last four to six days, starting heavier on days one and two (about eight tablespoons of blood), slowly tapering off the last few days (anywhere between two and six tablespoons of blood). Bleeding should not at any point be excessive, meaning you should be able to make it through a few hours with a super tampon and not leak. On the other end of the spectrum, if you need to wear only pantie liners when you have your period, even on days one and two, that's not normal. The blood should be a garnetlike fresh red color; it shouldn't be dark brown or pale pink. Small, wet Kleenex-tissue-like, dime-sized clots are considered normal; big quarter-sized ones are not.

One thing to remember when talking about your period is that in order for something to be considered problematic, it has to happen three months in a row. So if one month you get a period that is way out of sorts for you, definitely look back over the month and try to draw a correlation, but don't freak out.

Follow my advice in this book and see if your monthly PMS doesn't disappear.

· SEX DRIVE ·

Girl, you should want to have sex. Regularly. When you have sex, it shouldn't hurt internally (unless he is *that* well-endowed). You should be a raging horn dog when you are ovulating (which occurs at the midpoint of your monthly menstrual cycle, around day fourteen if you have a twenty-eight-day cycle). We are horn dogs when ovulating because we are dropping an egg that could potentially be made into a baby. At the most basic level we are animals and our body gets all hyped up at the thought of sperm when there is an eager egg ready and waiting. That's why when you are on the birth control pill, you have no sex drive. It shuts down ovulation. Get it?

Read more about ovulation and sex in chapters 7 and 9.

· VAGINAL DISCHARGE ·

The only time you should see vaginal discharge is during ovulation. This discharge, which is also known as cervical mucus, should show up as you approach ovulation. Ovulation occurs at the midpoint of a menstrual cycle, as I said above. If you have a twenty-eight-day cycle, then you should ovulate around day fourteen.

A few days before you ovulate (around day ten or eleven in a twenty-eight-day cycle), you should see a small amount of cervical mucus that is moist or sticky and white or cream in color. As you get closer to ovulation (days thirteen and fourteen), the amount of mucus will significantly increase and it will become very stretchy and egg-whitish looking. Right after ovulation (day fifteen) there is a marked change in mucus appearance; the amount diminishes and it gets sticky again. Within a day or two there should be no more mucus.

So, other than right around ovulation, you should not have vaginal discharge—a teeny, tiny amount of clear discharge the rest of the month can be considered normal. But if the amount of discharge requires you to wear a pantie liner, that's not normal. You should not see yellow, bloody or brown discharge at any point. There should not—at any time—be an odor coming from your vagina. The colorful, curdlike types of discharge are usually signs of an infection of sorts. Try some of the tips in chapter 9, take a probiotic—and see your gyno.

• SWEATING •

Sweat is normal with exertion. You shouldn't be sweating at night. You shouldn't have sweaty hands and feet. In CM, excessive sweating is usually a sign of weak Qi and a compromised immune system and most likely occurs in an overly anxious and nervous person.

Read about managing your stress in chapter 3. Read more about controlling anxiety and depression in chapter 4. And read more about controlling sweating in chapter 9.

• HEAD SPACE •

All right, we all have our bad days when we are irritable and cranky and can't stand anyone. But these days should be few and far between. For the most part, we should feel good and even-keeled. Not too low. Not too high. Just right. You shouldn't wake up with anxiety that lasts all day long. Or have palpitations that take your breath away. Nor should you wake up, on a regular basis, with zero desire to get out of bed. But for some reason, we do. In 2006 one in six American women between the ages of twenty-five and forty-four was prescribed an antidepressant medication. Ladies, what's going on? Why are we turning to medications to help us cope?

No worries, I'll teach you how to get a grip on your emotions in chapter 4. And you'll learn how to get a hold on your overwhelming stress in chapter 3. You can do it!

• ENERGY AND FOCUS-ABILITY •

If you are eating nutrient-rich food, metabolizing it properly and sleeping enough, you should have enough energy to get through your day. Of course, nobody is perfect and there will be days that we all feel draggy and listless, but for the most part, you should be able to make it through your day without the need for a caffeine or sugar boost. Seriously, you should be able to focus on tasks at hand and maintain a good level of concentration.

"But how? I can't make it through the afternoon without my second cup of coffee!"

Bottom line: if you can't focus and your energy is shot, you are not eating a good and balanced diet and/or you are not getting restorative sleep. I mean it!

You'll get plenty of information on improving your energy level and focus-ability throughout this entire book.

• SKIN, HAIR AND NAILS •

SHE'S GOT *THAT* GLOW

Your skin should shine and glow. Your cheeks should be naturally rosy. If your internal health is stellar, your skin will be the envy of all your girlfriends!

Your skin is an external manifestation of your internal health. According to CM,

- if it's dry—your insides are dehydrated and undernourished;
- if it's pimply—your insides are filled with phlegm and mucus;
- if it's red—your insides are hot and inflamed, or you are allergic to something in your diet or your environment;

- if it's excessively oily—your body is having a hard time metabolizing foods and is filled with phlegm (I'll tell you more about phlegm in chapter 5).

In your twenties and thirties, it is not normal to have dark circles under your eyes, puffy eyes, a ruddy complexion, rosacea or acne. Ladies, you are in your prime and you should have that youthful glow! Don't worry, I'll give you some great pointers on enhancing your inner and outer beauty in chapter 8.

RAPUNZEL-LIKE HAIR

Your hair, like your skin, is an external manifestation of your internal health. It should be lustrous and shiny and like Rapunzel's: magnificent and as fine as spun gold. Darlin', it shouldn't be falling out in clumps or going gray just yet.

According to the tenets of CM, our hair should begin to fall out around age thirty-five and it shouldn't go gray until we are forty-two! Going gray in your thirties is a sign of premature aging and doesn't say the best things about the state of your health.

Hair loss shows poor circulation, not enough Qi, a slow metabolism and a body low on vital reserves. Not good.

HARD AS NAILS

Your nails should grow. They should be thick and strong. They should not peel, crack or bend. If they do, you are not getting enough fat or nutrients from your diet. Or maybe you have a nail fungus. Women with a weak immune system have weak and brittle nails and can't fight off funky fungi.

Your cuticles should not be dry. If they are, you are dehydrated.

Read chapter 8 for more information on keeping your skin, hair and nails amazingly lustrous and fabulous all the time!

• • •

· TOO HOT, TOO COLD ·

Like Goldilocks, you shouldn't be too hot or too cold; you should be just right. Hormonal fluctuations can make us so hot at night that we peel off the covers and strip off our clothes; poor circulation will make our hands and feet as cold as ice. Neither should be the case. Of course it's normal to catch a chill once in a while or feel hot under the covers; these things are not normal, though, when they affect your quality of life.

When your body is properly nourished and you are getting enough exercise, your circulation shouldn't be impaired. When your hormones are balanced, you shouldn't have night sweats. Read more about balancing your hormones in chapter 7. Read more about maintaining a normal body temperature in chapter 9.

· HEADACHES ·

Headaches are not normal. Once in a while, sure. But as a general rule, headaches should not be a part of your life.

If headaches are ruining your days, you could be allergic to something you are eating or living with, you could be ingesting too much NutraSweet (or aspartame), you could have a hormonal imbalance, you could have poor circulation, or it could be a sinus infection or seasonal allergies. There are plenty of reasons for headaches. Advice for treating them can be found throughout this book, specifically in chapter 9. If you see that your headaches directly correlate with your menstrual cycle, follow my advice in chapter 7.

· BEING SICK SUCKS ·

It's normal to get sick once a year. Anything more than that shows a compromised immune system, deficient Qi and a weak body. It's not normal to get sick each month around your period.

When the seasons change, it is common to get a cold, but it isn't inevitable. If you have a strapping immune system (remember, daily banana-like bowel movements = strapping immune system), you should have ample Qi and be able to make it through the seasonal changes without getting laid up for a few days with a bad cold. Even if you work with a ton of peeps who are dragging in germs left and right, you should be able to ward them off. Ladies, germs are everywhere, all the time. It's not your exposure to them that gets you sick; it's your immune system's weakness.

Plenty of sleep + proper digestion of nutrient-rich foods = beautiful brown banana-like poop = > strapping immune system! Yay!

· PAIN ·

Nope, you shouldn't have any. We have a saying in Chinese Medicine that goes like this: If there is a free flow of energy (aka Qi), there is no pain. If energy (aka Qi) is not flowing freely, there is pain and disease will arise.

Energy—Qi—flows smoothly in a body that gets enough rest and exercise, efficiently digests its food and knows how to express its emotions.

· GIRL, BE MOD! ·

All right, now that I've completely convinced you that your body is ridiculously unhealthy, I want to give you another mantra to live by:

Everything in Moderation.

By this I mean, girl, BE MOD and don't freak out if on occasion you get gas or constipation, or have night sweats or a period one month that completely kicks your butt. It's when these symptoms are ever present that they indicate the overall state of your health is deteriorating. Shoot for your body functioning properly eighty to eighty-five percent of the time (that's five to six days a week); the other fifteen to twenty percent is margin for error.

Now we are going to get to the meat of the matter and get your internal and external health back into rock-solid shape so that it functions the way it should and you look and feel the best you've felt in ages. I'm going to show you the ropes so that you can fix the kinks in your system and avoid becoming that irritable, pill-popping, wrinkled, overweight and constipated old lady! All the information you need to get optimal health is in this book. Read it. Apply it. Live it. You will look younger, feel better and be sexy as hell. I know you can do it!

seriously, chill the F**k out!

$\mathcal{L}$ADIES, STRESS IS evil. Evil, evil, evil! We need to kick it in the butt and say, "Hit the road, Jack!"

Before I teach you how to do that, let's take a look at a couple of women who are just like you:

Meghan

AGE: Twenty-eight

JOB: Beauty editor

MEDICAL DIAGNOSIS: Irritable bowel syndrome

CHIEF COMPLAINT: Meghan wakes up every day extremely exhausted, bloated and anxious that her stomach will ruin yet another day at work. Regardless of what she eats, Meghan experiences unbearable symptoms of stomach cramping, diarrhea and nausea. The only correlation she has noticed is that the first "stomach attack" of the week occurs on Mondays, after she has lunch with her boss. These "stomach attacks" do not happen on vacation or over the weekends.

OTHER COMPLAINTS: Daily she is irritable and fatigued. She never feels she has enough energy to make it through the day. Premenstrually she experiences "outrageous bitchiness," severe lower-back cramping, skin breakouts and right-sided headaches.

MEDICATIONS: Imodium, Pepto-Bismol and Midol as needed (she is also considering the antidepressant Paxil, at the suggestion of her primary care physician).

Amanda

AGE: Thirty

JOB: Hedge fund analyst

MEDICAL DIAGNOSIS: Insomnia, TMJ, premature aging (deep facial wrinkles)

CHIEF COMPLAINT: On any given night Amanda doesn't get more than three hours of restless, jaw-clenched and dream-disturbed sleep. She also experiences night sweats that leave the back of her neck and her sheets drenched. This insomnia and TMJ have been going on since childhood, starting around the same time her parents divorced. If she wears her mouth guard (which would curtail the TMJ and clenching), she experiences horrible nightmares, so out of fear, she doesn't wear it.

OTHER COMPLAINTS: Anxiety, palpitations, deep facial wrinkles, fatigue, frequent and urgent urination, chronic urinary tract infections (UTIs), pain with sex due to vaginal dryness, dry scalp and heartburn.

MEDICATIONS: Xanax nightly and the occasional Unisom. Marijuana nightly. Yasmin (oral contraceptive). Antibiotics as needed for the UTIs. Zantac as needed. Her sleep doctor has recommended a nighttime combination of Ambien, Xanax and Paxil. Botox has been recommended for the wrinkles.

Now that you've read these two case studies, I'd like you to ask yourself the following questions. (Don't worry. This isn't really a quiz. I'll give you the answers!)

- Do I see myself in these women?
- What is the common denominator in these two cases?
- What is the Western recommended treatment for either case?

Answers: You are like these women (you did pick up this book, didn't you?), and stress (the common denominator) is making you anxious, wrinkly, bloated, sick and tired! And if left to the mere devices of Western medicine, you may wind up overmedicated and drug dependent by thirty-five!

Come on, I know you're smarter than that. I also know that today's woman is seriously overwhelmed. We are overworked over-achievers who are trying to sustain a "healthy" lifestyle as well as climb the ladder to success. We're not entirely succeeding. We are inundated with deadlines, the need for success and the desire to be perfect. We are seriously stressing the health out of ourselves.

Me included. Stress is around every corner, and if I'm not vigilant, it can get the best of my health too.

Stress usually comes up for me over work or money or boy issues or a family matter or because I spread myself way too thin schedulewise and I am running around like a maniac trying to please every single person in my life. When this happens, I usually lose sleep, I clench my jaw, my neck and shoulders ache with tension, I get constipated, I have vivid dreams and my eczema creeps up on my hands and my eyelids (making them red and itchy and puffy— it's über attractive!). Occasionally I'll get diarrhea too. Woo! Stress ROCKS! The only way I manage is to get out of my head and into my body and force myself to take a step back and prioritize. I call it Chilling the F**k Out.

Now, telling myself (or you) to Chill the F**k Out (CTFO) may sound harsh, but girls, I'm just trying to get your attention. And I'm not here to sugarcoat things (because as you all will know by the end of this book, sugar is evil). I am here to teach you, as I was taught, to draw the correlations between mind and body, to manage stress and to make CTFO-ing a top priority. For example, when you eat and then thirty minutes afterward you're on the bowl with di-arrhea, don't you think, WHAT THE HECK is wrong here? While you are sitting on the bowl waiting for the fun to stop, you should think, What is it that is stressing the shit out of me (literally)?

Darlin', this is serious business. It has recently been estimated that sixty to ninety percent of all doctors' visits are for a "stress-related" disorder. That means that most of the times we go to see the doctor, we are complaining about things such as insomnia, digestive prob-lems, muscular tension, headaches, palpitations, fatigue, infertility and menstrual disorders.

OK, ladies, it's officially gone too far.

Think about it, how many times has stress caused your period to be late, given you a horrible night's sleep, or left you vulnerable to that nasty bug going around the office? Or better yet, tell me if this has ever happened to you: you visit your doctor about an issue for which, after a barrage of tests, no known cause could be found, and he/she recommends that you consider taking an antidepressant? Did you ever get the feeling that your doctor was telling you, "These symptoms are all in your head"?

Hmmmm … sometimes I wonder the same. And I bet you do as well. That's probably why you are still reading this book. I know you get it. I know you know stress is the culprit in many of your dis-comforts, but you just don't know what to do about it. Neither do the other women who were prescribed an antidepressant drug last year—that's one in every six American women. Jeez Louise!

Drawing the correlation between stress and ill health doesn't re-quire a degree in rocket science. We get the fact that stress is making us sick. What we don't get is how to treat these stress-related dis-orders beyond medicating them. Band-Aiding a seemingly obscure ailment with medications (like taking Zoloft to manage a bad breakup, or Zantac to deal with too many Hershey's Kisses and mo-jitos, or Ambien to deal with our incessant late-night racing thoughts) doesn't get to the root of the issue. In Chinese Medicine we call this type of Band-Aiding a "branch" treatment, meaning you're treating only the symptoms, not the root cause of the issue (like the poor diet or the obsessive thinking or the low self-esteem). Taking a pill to deal with these kinds of health-care issues is absolute hogwash, and I know you know that!

Girls, in my best Scarlett O'Hara impersonation, I plead: as God is my witness, we desperately need to get a grip!

CTFO-ing will help us get that grip.

For over three thousand years, CM has been clinically applying the principles of CTFO to prevent disease and deter untimely aging (without the need for prescription medications).

And I'm here to help you implement CTFO coping mechanisms, because it's about time you took control of your stress!

Before I explain from a CM perspective how stress caused both Meghan's and Amanda's illnesses, let's talk a little bit about how Western medicine views stress.

I'm sure you know this, but let's go over it anyway. In Western medicine, stress comes down to our good ol' fight-or-flight response, in which both adrenaline and cortisol are released from our adrenal glands, located directly on top of our kidneys. Physiologically, our heart rate increases, the blood vessels under our skin constrict to prevent blood loss in case of injury, our pupils dilate so we can see better and our blood sugar ramps up, giving us an energy boost. Once upon a prehistoric time we needed this fight-or-flight response to run from lions and tigers and bears or to stand and fight them. Now we use it to react to our jobs, our boyfriends, our scales, our moms and possibly our bare ring finger! And chronic stress, the kind we're under on a daily basis, now, that's a killer!

The stress response is in place to protect and support us. It's a *good* thing that when faced with a threat the body kicks into high gear to prepare for emergency action, enabling us to move and think faster, hit harder, see better, hear more acutely and jump higher. So, sure, stress is healthy, in MODERATION.

The problems occur when the stress cascade is activated repeatedly, hour after hour, deadline after deadline and chaotic moment after chaotic moment, rather than, say, once every few days when the lion came to your cave and stole your dinner. You see, the more the stress cascade is activated, the harder it is to shut it off. Instead of the body chilling out once the crisis has passed, your stress hormones, heart rate and blood pressure remain elevated (because the body hasn't had ample time to filter out the excess adrenaline and cortisol). This extended and repeated activation of the stress response takes a heavy toll on the body. The physical wear and tear it causes includes damage to the cardiovascular system and immune system suppression. Stress causes you to age prematurely, as in Amanda's deep facial lines. Stress compromises your ability to fight off disease, to get pregnant, to properly digest food, to flush out cellular toxins (that will cause cellulite and pimples), to get rid of abdominal fat and to sleep. And get this: excessive stress has been shown to stunt growth in children! It can even rewire the brain, leaving you more vulnerable to everyday pressures and mental-health problems such as anxiety and depression.

Now we get why all those women are taking drugs to deal!

How Acupuncture Relieves Stress

From a scientific perspective, acupuncture works to knock out stress by causing your body to release natural painkilling brain chemicals called endorphins. It also improves circulation, which oxygenates tissues and helps flush out excess adrenaline and cortisol (remember, those are the two major stress hormones), which cause stress to age us and make us sick. From a CM perspective, acupuncture improves the Qi and blood flow within the body, relieving the disease-causing tension and stagnation that is caused by stress. And on top of all that, acupuncture is oh-so-calming. It slows down your heart rate, lowers your blood pressure and relaxes your muscles.

Needle me, baby!

As if there wasn't enough proof that stress is evil, several groups of scientists have taken to researching the effects of stress on health.

Numerous studies have demonstrated a link between chronic stress and indexes of poor health, including risk factors for cardiovascular disease and poorer immune function. More recently, scientists at the University of California, San Francisco, have found that both perceived stress and chronic stress cause us to age at the cellular level (which means stress is causing our DNA, aka genes, to physically change!). As the authors concluded from their studies, "These findings have implications for understanding how, at the cellular level, stress may promote earlier onset of age-related diseases."

Stress affects us at the cellular level! It actually speeds the process of genetic and cellular degradation that leads to untimely aging and illness. When genes degrade, they split apart, causing systems to break down and reckless oxidation to ravage the body. Remember all that talk of antioxidants and how they fight aging? Well, it's this reckless oxidation that those antioxidants are trying to fight off. But when we are under chronic everyday stress—I don't care how many blueberries or goji berries you ingest—you ain't gonna win the battle. Oxidation will win and you will age and get sick. So what else can you do? Well, girls, I'm here to tell ya that the old-school Oriental CTFO approach is one of the best antioxidants on the market!

CM views stress similarly to Western science; we just use different language to describe it. You see, in CM, stress = chaos. And chaos = disorder and frenzied madness! Too much chaos and chronic stress cause all systems to function on overdrive, draining us of our precious Qi, and most important, stress seriously affects two organs: the kidneys and the liver. Basically, the liver gets really, really irritated and the kidneys get tired.

In CM, the liver is responsible for circulating blood and Qi and cleansing our body of emotional toxins like repressed anger, and environmental toxins like smog, nonorganic pesticide-ridden foods, mojitos, marijuana, excess hormones and bad cholesterol. But when we get stressed, the whole body gets tense, and liver circulation is hampered. The liver in turn gets backed up and unable to perform its job, making our internals an emotional and environmental toxic wasteland. A toxic woman is a sleep-deprived, bitchy and anxious one with outrageous PMS symptoms, excess abdominal fat and pimples (sounds like both Meghan and Amanda).

And then there are the kidneys. . . . In CM, the kidneys are our foundation; they are the source of our vitality; they are, as ancient CM texts proclaim, "the initial sprout of physical life." The kidneys store what we call "essence," or *jing*. "Essence," which could be loosely translated in Western terms as "genetic predisposition," is one of the three treasures of Traditional Chinese Medicine (the other two being our Qi and our spirit) and is the material basis for our physical bodies. We are each born with a certain amount of essence, which is given to us from our parents (our genes), and it's meant to last us our whole lives. In fact, the amount of essence we are born with determines how long we will live and the health in which we will live (and also our ability to have children). You could look at this essence as a bottle of La Prairie eye cream; you want to use only a very teeny tiny amount of it on a daily basis. At two hundred dollars an ounce, you'd never take it and liberally spread it on your thighs! Instead you'd use it sparingly, treating it like the precious substance it is. So when you think of essence, think of ridiculously expensive eye cream.

But here's the good news:

You can actually build essence!

It's almost like you can actually shift your genetic predispositions. You do this by eating healthfully, living peacefully, sleeping enough and expressing your emotions. By the same token, you can burn up this essence. Too much stress at work (like the kind that causes Meghan to poop her brains out), or partying, eating unhealthfully and harboring resentment or anger (like Amanda the insomniac), will use up this essence before it was meant to be used up. In all individuals, essence declines as we age. That's just the plain ol' truth. And as essence declines, we get weak and frail, we wrinkle, we become infertile, our hair grays and we're more susceptible to disease and illness. But what CM says is, you can use less essence each and every day if you treat your body properly. So think of it like this: if you eat well and sleep well and live a balanced and peaceful life, you'll be less toxic and need less of that overpriced eye cream. You'll always use it, but one bottle will last you longer than your counterpart who's out "burning the candle" (or should I say essence) at both ends. She'll wrinkle faster than you, get sick more often and have cellulite in godforsaken places. Not to mention she'll probably have a really hard time getting pregnant. Oh no!

So we now understand that when Meghan has to race to the bathroom after lunch with her boss, it's due to the fact that her liver is really tense and stagnant. Her work-related stress is causing her liver to cramp up and spit out bowel movements in the form of diarrhea. If this issue isn't resolved for Meghan, her body will eventually become malnourished (because her body doesn't have time to digest the food she eats; all it has time for is managing her overwhelming stress) and the kidneys will have to start using up her saved-up essence to help her get by because she has no good, clean Qi coming into her system. And voilà: she's exhausted, bloated and aging before her time!

In Amanda's case the liver is so pissed off and stagnant (and has been for some time), it actually begins to smolder, causing her body to overheat. This excess heat in her body both dehydrates her (causing premature wrinkles and dry skin) and manifests in symptoms such as anxiety, insomnia and heartburn (when there is a burning sensation in our bodies as in heartburn, CM sees this as too much internal heat—pretty logical, huh?). Picture it this way: the stress piles up like organic waste in a compost pile. As the pile sits longer and longer, it actually begins to smolder and decompose the organic matter. Amanda's stress is basically decomposing her insides. YUCK!!! If she doesn't stop the cycle now, she will most likely use up the majority of her stored essence just to get through her thirties and she'll get sicker and sicker in her forties. Not to mention all the antiaging creams she'll have to buy.

As you can see, dietary, physical and mental stress robs your kidneys of their essence and makes the liver toxic and tense. Chronic stress ages the bajeezus out of us (as kidney essence declines) and makes us sick (as liver function slows down and dirty nasty toxins build up in your body). The end result: a prematurely wrinkled, anxious, bloated, irritable, infertile, hormonally imbalanced and cellulite-filled insomniac who has to dye her hair because it's gone gray! Oh, and she'll be broke from spending all her money on anti-aging products and over-the-counter medicines!

If you are fine with all that, then rock on with your bad self. But I get the feeling you're smarter than that. So if you'd like to take back control from the evil demon called chronic stress, then read on, because I'll show you how to seriously Chill the F**k Out and challenge the damage of the massive stress meltdown.

· HOW TO CTFO AND · SHOW STRESS THE DOOR

How can we manage our stress and, more important, head off the damage that stress is doing? First, we must realize the physical and emotional impact stress has on us. Second, we must identify the stressors, and learn how to manage the necessary ones and get rid of the unnecessary ones. And then third, we get to tell stress (and our stressed-out selves) to CTFO!

Task 1:
RECOGNIZING THE PHYSICAL AND EMOTIONAL IMPACT STRESS HAS ON OUR BODIES

At this point I hope you are clear on the fact that stress ages the heck and the health out of us and we need to show it the door. With this first task, we are going to find out how bad it really is. Grab your pens ... and put on your most honest face. Following is an obnoxious list of all the big, bad, scary emotional and physical bummers stress can cause. I want you to make a check in the box next to any of the symptoms you currently experience on a weekly basis (so even if you have a symptom only once a week, check it off). Some symptoms may be present only the week before your period; write a P next to these symptoms.

Girl, do yourself a favor and be as honest with yourself as possible:

❑ Memory problems

❑ Inability to concentrate

❑ Seeing only the negative

❑ Poor judgment

❑ Feeling moody and hypersensitive

❑ Depression

❑ Feeling easily irritated and "on edge"

❑ Lack of confidence

❑ Headaches

❑ Muscle tension and pain

❑ Fatigue

❑ High blood pressure

❑ Asthma or shortness of breath

❑ Decreased sex drive

❑ Infertility

❑ Difficulty making decisions

❑ Confusion

❑ Repetitive or racing thoughts

❑ Desire to escape or run away

❑ Restlessness and anxiety

❑ Anger and resentment

❑ Sense of being overwhelmed

❑ Urge to laugh or cry at inappropriate times

❑ Digestive problems

❑ Sleep disturbances

❑ Chest pain, irregular heartbeat

❑ Weight gain or loss

❑ Skin problems

❑ Eating more or less

❑ PMS (even if you think it's normal)

☐ Sleeping too much or too little

☐ Panic attacks or panicky feelings

☐ Teeth grinding / jaw clenching

☐ Nervous habits (i.e., nail biting, pacing)

☐ Losing your temper

☐ Overreacting to unexpected problems

Now I'd like you to count up how many of the above symptoms you checked off. Write the number down here: _____.

Here, note how many P symptoms you checked off: _____.

And now for the scoring part.

If you checked

- **1–8:** Yay! Good for you! You're doing all right, but CTFO-ing anyway can't hurt and it'll help you fight the aging process.
- **9–18:** Eh, you could use a little help; stress is definitely affecting you more than you think.
- **19–27:** Oh dear, you need to CTFO regularly. Stress has got you by the balls.
- **28–36:** You seriously need to CTFO ALL THE TIME. WE MAY NEED TO ADMIT YOU TO A CTFO CLINIC.

Now, if you checked off eight or more P symptoms, your liver is officially toxic and tense. But don't worry, there is hope for you yet. (For more-specific help with managing your PMS, apply what I say in chapter 7.)

So tell me, girl, after looking over these lists, how stressed are you? I mean, in all honesty, you picked up this book, and you've read this far; you must be aware that something isn't right!

If you see yourself in these symptoms, it is my job to remind you that you need to take some control back. You need to use the tools that I offer to combat stress and the resulting poor health and untimely aging.

Mayday, Mayday!

If, in addition to a plethora of symptoms we just went through, you experience any of the following stress-induced scenarios (again, honesty is expected!) with some level of frequency, we definitely need you to CTFO, but it's also highly recommended that you get some T-time! No, I am not talking golf; I am talking therapy. Unfortunately stress has got you good and you need more than this book; you need some professional mental help:

- Isolating yourself from others
- Neglecting your responsibilities
- Increasing alcohol and drug use
- Overdoing activities such as exercising or shopping

Task 2:
IDENTIFYING THE STRESSORS

Listen, if we identify our stressors, we can effectively prepare ourselves to deal with them. Moreover, if we organize and prioritize our stressors, we can really get a grip on them.

"Organize and prioritize my stress, Aimee?"

Yes! Let's figure out which ones are important, which ones are imaginary and which ones are out of our control. Seriously, a lot of our stressors are completely and totally out of our control. We have to learn to let go of stressing over nonsensical issues such as death or unborn children or the lack of your soul mate or other people's approval or disapproval. We cannot control other people, nor can we control life's uncertainties. Stop trying! Control your health instead.

Make each day the best it can be. Make each day feel the best it can feel. And do this all while treating yourself right and looking better. Do this by prioritizing your health. And I'm not talking just about going to the gym. I'm talking about mental health, dietary health and conscious health. Girl, you have got to get a grip and take back some control. Don't let this crazy demon called chronic stress ruin your health!

All right, let's organize and prioritize your stressors. We are going to make a list. Get yourself a piece of paper and make four columns on it.

The first column is labeled STRESS. In this column, list the things that bring you stress in your daily life. For example, work, significant other, family, friends, chores such as going to the gym or food shopping, managing your finances, managing your weight, eating healthy, trying to get pregnant, insomnia, anxiety, daily commuting.

The second column is labeled HAPPY/GRATEFUL. In this column, write down the things in your current life that make you happy and grateful. Not things that you think will make you happy, but things that actually do make you happy. For example, friends, work (believe it or not, some people actually enjoy their jobs), the ability to pay your bills on time, healthy bowel movements, your significant other, exercise, hobbies, meditation. You get the idea, right?

The third column is labeled BALANCE. Beneath this heading I want you to write the things that currently bring balance or peace or calm to your daily life. But here you can also put things that you think could bring you peace in your daily life (i.e., things you've thought about doing, or things you have done in the past but never get around to doing anymore).

Some things may appear in more than one column. That's fine. But really spend time on this. I want you to have at least ten things listed in each column. You can do it!

Work on these three columns first before moving on to the fourth column.

The fourth column is labeled PRIORITY. And in this column write down everything you listed in the other three columns in order, from the items you give the most importance to in your daily life to those that you give the least importance to. What do you spend the most time doing? What takes up the most physical energy? What takes up the most emotional energy? Again, spend some good quality time on this. Focus and be honest with yourself. This way you can fix yourself.

After you are done, look at this priority list carefully. How high up do your *HAPPY/GRATEFUL* and *BALANCE* items fall? Are all your top priorities your main stressors? Does meditation or healthy eating fall anywhere on ANY of the lists? Is exercise causing you more stress or more happiness? When you exercise, are you thinking about work? How about your sleep—is it peaceful or roiled by worries and crazy vivid dreams? Or are you an insomniac who knows that while the rest of the world is peacefully sleeping, you'll be up all night, fitfully floundering?

Now we have to figure out how we can make some of the things that make you happy and balanced top priority rather than low man on the totem pole. And how we can eradicate from your list some of the crap that stresses you out. What are you willing to give up? Maybe if you didn't have that second glass of wine last night, you'd have the energy to get up early and hit the gym? Or how about adding to your weekly task list of chores things like "Turn off cell phone at nine p.m. Monday through Wednesday," "Take a deep breath" or "Cook myself a hundred percent organic meal"? Here's another idea: flip your list. Make your last priority first and your first, last. See how that makes you feel.

"All right," you say, "I get it: stress is the almighty evil of all evils. It's bad, bad, bad. But tell me, how do I deal with it? I can't quit my job. I can't tell my boss to shove it up her you know what. I can't stop paying my bills or ignore my needy friends. How do I manage all my stressors?"

Denise, one of my best friends, called me one Sunday night. She felt she was having a panic attack. Her upcoming week was jam-packed with work dinners, year-end reports were due, her mom was being a bitch and her period was late.

After listening to her reel off all her issues, and convincing her she shouldn't quit her job nor break up with her mom, I said to her, "You need to Chill the F**k Out."

I e-mailed her this chapter (the one you're reading right now) and told her to give it a good, hard, knock-some-sense-into-yourself read. She did.

She e-mailed me about an hour later, telling me that she checked off thirty of the boxes on the checklist! The realization that stress was compromising her health made her more anxious at first (especially because she didn't have time in her schedule to check into a CTFO clinic!). When she got to task two and made her lists, she realized that there were few things she did in her life that made her happy. She realized work was her top priority. She told me that when she read the part where I wrote, "I mean, really, is it necessary to keep up with the latest headline news every night?" she felt liberated, like I had just given her permission to turn off CNN.

After she turned off CNN, she took a much-needed CTFO break and had herself a good cry.

The next day she sent me her first grati-text, "I am grateful for my CTFO time."

Now we send grati-texts to each other every day.

First, you prioritize happiness (move one of the items on your HAPPY/GRATEFUL list to the top of your priority list) and create space for balance and peace in your life (again, make one or two items from your list a priority). You will better manage your stress by prioritizing happiness and balance.

Second, you can further organize your stressors and teach yourself to stop worrying about the things you have no control over (like whether it's going to rain the day you want to wear your new open-toed flats). In order to do this, you must pick and choose your battles with vigilance. By prioritizing and being selective, you can streamline your life. Honestly ask yourself what you can really, TRULY handle, what you really need to do on your to-do list. I mean, really, is it necessary to keep up with the latest headline news every night? Or to have your sock drawer organized by color? Or are you actually making yourself more stressed? Rather, learn to focus on that which is essential to your health and well-being (like things that make you feel happy and balanced) and minimize all the other BS. How about turning off the TV, computer and BlackBerry and silencing the phone by a certain time every night? It's like you're back in summer camp and it's "lights out" time. Seriously, try it for one month. I guarantee you'll be more relaxed and have a more peaceful sleep. Sure, at first this process may make you feel a bit more anxious, but that will subside. CTFO living requires perseverance! You can do it!

Third, you give yourself daily "CTFO time"!

"How do I do that, Aimee?"

Let's discuss.

Task 3:
CHILL THE F**K OUT—ON A DAILY BASIS

When you CTFO daily, you give yourself some much-needed downtime. When you prioritize "CTFO time," you are less stressed and more healthy.

Teach me, already!

Ladies, CTFO time is an easy five-to-ten-minute break. This is what you have to do:

- Find yourself a secluded and quiet place. At home this may be the living room couch or your bedroom. At work this could be your office, the bathroom or outside (those cigarette smokers get outside—why can't you?).
- Turn off things like the ringer on your cell phone or Black-Berry so that they cannot interrupt you.
- Set the alarm on your phone (or computer or alarm clock) for five to ten minutes (or for however long you want to CTFO).
- Sitting comfortably, with your shoulders dropped and your jaw and fists relaxed, rest your hands on your lap, palms up toward the sky.

- Close your eyes or fix them on something, such as a picture on the wall.
- Breathe. This breathing is the deep, deeeeeep-breathing kind. I want you to breathe so deeply that your belly rises. The breathing cycle should be a deep breath in (three to four seconds), belly rise, hold for a count of two seconds, then a long slow exhale (again, three to four seconds). For the first couple of times try resting one of your hands on your abdomen so that you feel it rise and fall with each breath. Nice and slowly.
- Try using one of my guided-imagery CTFO times that can be downloaded to your iPod from my Web site, www.aimeeraupp.com.

Now, I'm not saying that while you are sitting there breathing and CTFO-ing, thoughts of work or life or stress won't enter your mind; they will, there's no doubt about that. Just do your best to let them come into your mind and then pass through, and just keep breathing. I am also not saying this will be easy at first. It will take time. Remember, to CTFO requires perseverance! You can do it! Figure on having five restless CTFO sessions before you have a peaceful one. But keep at it. It's so rewarding AND it breaks that damn stress cycle. Breaking the stress cycle a few times each day makes you healthier, with more essence and less toxic liver tension. Put another way, getting you to CTFO will fight aging and disease!

And, if you're feeling really zealous, I recommend you incorporate the following sixteen-minute rockin', stress-busting CTFO regimen into your day:

- Take three minutes each morning to journal your feelings, thoughts and physical symptoms. This is a great way to get in touch with the stranger known as yourself! (Learn more about journaling in chapter 4.)
- Allow for five to ten minutes of CTFO time twice a day— once in the morning and once in the afternoon or evening.

- Before bed take three minutes (or more, if you feel like it) and write down the things that are on your mind. Look at this ritual as one that takes your thoughts out of your head and puts them on a piece of paper. This allows you to decide to let those things go so that you can get a good night's sleep and have the energy to tackle your tasks tomorrow.

Now, before you start kvetching, "Aimee, I don't have time to CTFO for five minutes, let alone time for this sixteen-minute regimen, ugh!" listen very closely to what I have to say (go ahead, put your ear to the page): SUCK IT UP! Stress will age you and make you sick! Acknowledge the fact that your health will suffer, and you will wrinkle before your time and spend loads of money on antiaging products that work only on the superficial level.

Listen, your stress needs to be managed so that its damage can be prevented. And really, it's not that hard. I mean, what is sixteen minutes? Eight minutes in the morning, eight minutes in the evening. That's nothing, man.

If people take unhealthy cigarette breaks, you can certainly take your CTFO time. The world will not end if you take a five- or ten-minute reprieve from the office chaos, a walk outside the building, a rest on the john or a sip of tea in the kitchen. In Aimee's perfect world, cigarettes wouldn't exist and every office would make CTFO time mandatory.

Now, to reiterate, you have to make this a habit! You will not reap the benefits of CTFO time overnight. Like anything else, this is a process and it requires persistence. You need to do this once or twice a day, every day. For me it works best when I do my first one in the morning at home; this way I feel nice and balanced at the start of my day. Then I try for my second whenever I can sneak the time. Sure, there are days that I can't get that second one in, but I try.

Incorporating daily CTFO time will chill you the f**k out, and it will seriously allow you to tackle the everyday challenges that will inevitably be there. Women who CTFO on a regular basis are not as bitchy and have less anxiety, better digestion, stronger immune systems, glowing skin and healthier relationships. What are you waiting for? Madonna and Jen Aniston meditate, shouldn't you? I do it and you can too!

Task 4:
BEING HAPPY WITH WHAT YOU'VE GOT

Ladies, true happiness is created gradually and does not come in the form of the hottest handbag. When you are happy, life is just better. Quit waiting for some lover (or baby or new job or more money) to come into your life and make you happy. If you are not happy now, nothing is gonna change that except YOU. We can always daydream about the things that we need, or the person that we need, to make us happier. But that's so not you and you know it. Do things for yourself that make you happy, from the inside out.

A constant longing for things outside of your present situation creates an endless cycle of unhappiness and is unsettling to your spirit. True happiness starts with acceptance of self and what you have right now. What makes you happy? You don't know? Go back to that HAPPY/GRATEFUL list and think about the things that you are grateful for in your life, things that you have RIGHT NOW, RIGHT HERE that make you happy or grateful. Spend time with this. If you don't feel you have happiness in your life, create it!

Task 5:
CREATING HAPPINESS

Having a hard time being happy with what you've got? Well, then, let's create some happiness!

Try the following:

- **GRATI-TEXT.** Find a friend to do "gratitude" work with. Each morning e-mail or text each other with one thing in your life you are grateful for. It can be as simple as "I just had the best night's sleep. I am grateful for that." Or "I am grateful for the ability to pay my bills on time." You get it, right? Do this every day for a couple of months and see your life change. I am serious. Focus on the positive; make happiness and gratitude a larger part of your life.

- **FAKE IT TILL YOU MAKE IT.** Another way to create happiness is what my mother calls "Fake it till you make it." Go on, pretend you're happy; fake happiness until you find it. Like attracts like, and happiness—even if it's all an act—will attract happiness into your life. Do it. Put on a happy face and walk down the street. Come on, girl, you can do it. Happiness can be yours.

"I don't feel like faking happiness, Aimee!"

Why not? You have nothing to lose and you won't just attract happiness into your life; you'll get healthier too!

Ladies, happy people are healthier than unhappy ones. In fact, psychology researchers at Carnegie Mellon University concluded from scientific study that "happiness and other positive emotions play an even more important role in health than previously thought." It's no wonder; happier people create happiness around them and like attracts like. If we are happy (truly happy), we will attract only happy and positive things to our lives, not ill health! And another thing: happy people have more sex than unhappy ones! So come on, girls, make your life happy and have more sex!

Other things you can do to create happiness: cook yourself an amazing dinner, fill up your fruit bowl with fresh organic fruits, decorate your home with plants and candles, create a nice cozy CTFO space in your place, focus on the things in your life that already bring you happiness and gratitude and do them more. And most important, prioritize happiness! Or just fake it till you make it, because you deserve to be happy. Come on, girl, I know you can do it!

mental Detox

$\mathcal{A}$LYSSA, A THIRTY-FIVE-YEAR-OLD flourishing interior designer, came to me panicky and distressed after a recent broken engagement. Her fiancé was cheating on her. Argh! She couldn't sleep and of course she was having incessant, racing, fear-provoking am-I-going-to-be-single-forever thoughts over the big breakup. Her primary care physician had prescribed Zoloft for her symptoms. She came to me hoping to manage her insomnia and anxiety "naturally" without medications; she was also really put off that her doctor didn't offer her any other means of dealing with her anxiety. I empathized. Rather than recommending lifestyle approaches like meditation, journaling, therapy or kicking a punching bag with her ex's face on it to help her through her heartache, her doctor gave her a pill to dull her feelings. She's not alone.

One in six American women between the ages of twenty-five and forty-four was prescribed an antidepressant like Zoloft, Celexa, Wellbutrin and Paxil in 2006.

Listen, I understand that most of us need help with managing our emotions. And for many people, antidepressants are a lifesaver, as mental illnesses are serious and very real. But the thing to keep in mind is that diagnosing a mental illness (and deciding to medicate a mental illness) should never be done lightly and must involve not only a physician but a psychiatric evaluation. Unfortunately, our Western culture is Speedy Gonzales quick to medicate without a clear-cut mental-illness diagnosis, leaving so many in the affect-dulled dark as to the root causes of their emotional and physical symptoms. This rash, let's-medicate-your-blues-away approach leads to a very unhealthy level of emotional repression, discouraging you from expressing and exploring your emotions and the stressors behind them. Girl, you've got to learn to feel your emotions, each and every emotion, each and every day. And girl, you have GOT to learn to express yourself! Before swallowing that pill, try recognizing the emotions—both good and bad—that you feel from moment to moment, and realize that they are a major thread in your human spirit. Before swallowing that pill, inspect your daily coping mechanisms and try the lifestyle approaches I encourage in this book (particularly in this chapter) to decrease and manage your symptoms naturally. Ladies, medication should be the LAST resort, not the first.

The two most common emotional issues for which drugs are prescribed to the thirty-something-year-old woman are anxiety and depression; usually they coexist. Let's quickly run through the Western diagnostics of these two mental illnesses. Watch out, I'm about to put on my "serious cap" for a couple of moments because these mental illnesses are very real and their symptoms should never be ignored.

· DEPRESSION ·

Clinical depression is unrelenting and overwhelming. Those suffering from depression often describe it as "living in a black hole" or an unshakable feeling of doom. Clinically depressed individuals can't escape their unhappiness and despair. They often feel lifeless, empty and unable to experience any sort of pleasure. Not even a great new Gucci handbag can shake their gloom.

Individuals with depression will not present with every symptom (see box), and the severity of symptoms can vary widely from person to person. The key, however, is that the symptoms must **persist DAILY for at least two weeks** before being considered a potential sign of clinical depression, unless of course there are suicidal thoughts or attempts.

Some Symptoms of Clinical Depression

- Persistent sadness, anxiety and/or "blue" mood
- Loss of appetite and/or weight loss, or overeating and/or weight gain
- Insomnia or the desire to sleep a lot
- Restlessness and/or irritability
- Feelings of worthlessness, inappropriate guilt and/or helplessness
- Feelings of hopelessness
- Difficulty thinking, concentrating and/or making decisions
- Thoughts of death or suicide and/or attempts at suicide
- Loss of interest or pleasure in hobbies and activities that you once enjoyed
- Withdrawal from social situations, family and friends
- Decreased energy, fatigue and overall lethargic feeling
- Persistent physical symptoms like headaches, digestive problems and pain

Before a diagnosis of depression is made, a physician should perform a complete medical exam (ruling out possible physical illnesses like hypothyroidism that can cause symptoms of depression), and a detailed psychological evaluation should be done by a physician, psychiatrist or psychologist. Your primary care physician or your dentist should not prescribe an antidepressant to you just because you tell him you are stressed-out and having diarrhea. Get it?

We've all been depressed with a lowercase d, where we call up our mothers or our best friends and say with a sigh, "I'm depressed." We feel down, we cry at commercials and we want nothing more than to stay in bed all day and feel sorry for ourselves. But these symptoms usually pass and can typically be rectified by a good laugh or an hour of exercise. This is NOT clinical depression. It is a transient depressed state, but it is not despair or doom. The same goes for the depression we've all experienced after a bad breakup; you can't eat, you can't sleep and you cry in the middle of the supermarket when you see his favorite cereal, but this is NOT clinical depression even if it lasts weeks or months (in some people a precipitating event like a bad breakup can trigger clinical depression, but that's not typical).

· ANXIETY ·

There are quite a few anxiety disorders (see box on the following page). The key thing to remember about anxiety disorders is that a clinical diagnosis should technically be made only after a person is experiencing symptoms **DAILY for at least six months**. And diagnosis must be made through a detailed psychological evaluation by a physician, psychiatrist or psychologist. Period.

Symptoms that may also be part of the daily presentation of an anxiety disorder are fatigue, trembling, restlessness, palpitations, muscle tension, shortness of breath, rapid heart rate, dry mouth, cold hands, headaches, diarrhea, insomnia, nausea, grinding of teeth, dizziness, feeling keyed up, irritability, increased startling and impaired concentration. Again, these symptoms should be present daily for AT LEAST six months before a psychiatric diagnosis and medication are technically warranted (unless there are suicidal thoughts or tendencies or paranoid and delusional behavoir).

Girl, from the moment you start feeling the symptoms of anxiety, you can do so many things that will help your condition naturally.

Types of Anxiety Disorders

- **Generalized anxiety disorder (GAD).** GAD is characterized by constant worrying and fear that distract you from your day-to-day activities or a persistent feeling that something bad is going to happen. People with GAD feel anxious almost all the time.

- **Obsessive-compulsive disorder (OCD).** OCD is characterized by unwanted thoughts or behaviors that seem impossible to stop or control. You may be troubled by obsessions, such as a recurring worry that you forgot to turn off the oven or the iron. You may also suffer from uncontrollable compulsions, such as washing your hands over and over or having to do activities in a specific order.

- **Panic attacks and panic disorder.** Panic disorder is characterized by repeated, unexpected panic attacks that can last up to thirty minutes. Panic disorder may also be accompanied by agoraphobia, which is a fear of being in places where escape or help would be difficult in the event of a panic attack. If you have agoraphobia, you are likely to avoid public places such as shopping malls or confined spaces such as an airplane or an elevator.

- **Phobias.** Phobia is characterized by an unrealistic or exaggerated fear of a specific object, activity or situation that in reality presents little to no danger.

- **Separation anxiety.** Separation anxiety is a normal part of child development. It consists of crying and distress when a child is separated from a parent or away from home. If separation anxiety persists beyond a certain age or interferes with daily activities, it can be a sign of separation anxiety disorder.

- **Social anxiety/social phobia.** This is characterized by a debilitating fear of being seen negatively by others and humiliated in public.

Don't get me wrong—if you feel like hurting yourself or frequently behave in a self-destructive fashion, like drinking your face off every night or blowing off work, medication may be necessary (and therapy mandatory). But that pill, if necessary, should not be a permanent fixture in your life. Instead it should serve as a means to an end while you learn to implement lifestyle tools to help get your life back on track.

Certainly there are people who have true chemical imbalances and require a lifetime of medication. Most of us don't. The bottom line is, it is imperative that you get a complete psychiatric evaluation and receive a firm diagnosis before making a decision about taking an antidepressant or an antianxiety medication.

Transient episodes of anxiety, like the ones that happen before a big work presentation or a first date, are definitely not worthy of medication. You should not need to take a Xanax to get through a big day. You can calm yourself without medicines. I will show you how.

· CHINESE MEDICINE AND THE · MIND-BODY CONNECTION

In Chinese Medicine, the body and the mind are interconnected. The body creates the energy for the mind to function rationally. The mind is the expression of the body's ability to properly manufacture energy from the foods we eat, how much we sleep and the way we manage our stress. Therefore, according to CM theory, when your body is unhealthy, so is your mind and vice versa. And it is harmful to the body when the mind's emotional states are masked by prescription medications, your vice of choice or plain old ignorance, because suppressing your emotions will negatively affect your physical health, causing wrinkles, constipation, dark under-eye circles, insomnia and infertility!

"Wait, Aimee, did you just say that ignoring my emotions can cause infertility too?"

Seems like everything you've read about so far in this book

causes infertility, doesn't it? I hope you're beginning to see a pattern: if you're a thirty-something-year-old woman, being reckless not only with your physical health but with your mental health will make it harder for you to have babies. Let me explain. Repressing your emotional experiences, whether it be by taking medication, drinking a cocktail or simply ignoring how you feel, will have negative repercussions on all your internal organs, primarily your liver. We talked about the liver quite a bit in chapter 3; to recap, in CM theory the liver is the organ largely responsible for circulating blood and Qi throughout the body, managing the menstrual cycle, detoxifying the whole body and maintaining emotional stability. When you mask your emotional state (much the same as when you are stressed to the max, don't eat healthfully, have poor digestion or don't exercise or sleep enough), your liver gets pissed off because it can't do its job, and it becomes dysfunctional. A dysfunctional liver has a hard time maintaining a normal menstrual cycle, and a woman with abnormal menstruation probably isn't ovulating regularly and will have a hard time getting pregnant. Make sense?

An irregular menstrual cycle is just one of the bad things that can happen when our emotions are repressed and our liver becomes stagnant and dysfunctional. The big scary one is a toxic liver. We've all heard about "detox diets" and have read in a gazillion magazines what to eat to detox your liver. You've also heard somewhere (for one, in this book) that a toxic liver will lead to premature aging, wrinkles, acne, cellulite, excess abdominal fat and a higher likelihood of getting really sick with illnesses like high cholesterol, diabetes, thyroid disease, cancer and infertility.

Unfortunately, these detox discussions always leave out this pearl of information: any emotion when unchecked will be toxic to your liver too.

Let's break it down further.

In CM, we recognize seven major emotional states: joy, worry (or overthinking), anxiety, anger, sorrow, fear and terror (which is like fear on crack—fear is "Sure, I'm fearful, but I'll give it a shot"; terror is "No freaking way, I'm not doing it!"). All these emotional states are natural and normal when experienced appropriately (like when you get angry with your dry cleaner for losing your favorite white Theory pants) but not excessively (OK, you're mad at Mr. Dry Cleaner, but there's no need to give him dirty looks every time you see him). It's when these emotions—any of them, even joy—become excessive that health issues will arise.

"Wait, too much joy can make me sick and toxic?"

Yes. Each emotion elicits a physical reaction. Try this: think of a joyful memory, like kissing the first love of your life. How did you physically feel? You probably felt butterflies in your tummy and a pulsing in the center of your chest. Joy is a high; physiologically it's an adrenaline rush. Now imagine feeling like that ALL THE TIME. It'd feel uncomfortable, right? Too much joy will eventually cause mania, restlessness, nonstop palpitations; it'll tax the shit out of your adrenal glands the same way chronic stress does. And if you remember from chapter 3, chronic stress has been scientifically proven to promote an earlier onset of age-related diseases like heart disease, diabetes, thyroid disease and high cholesterol. Sounds the same as the toxic-liver list, doesn't it?

Let's do another exercise: I want you to remember the last time you felt anger. Maybe it was yesterday when a coworker pissed you off. Do you remember what physically happened? Chances are your jaw clenched and your whole body became rigid with tension, especially your neck and shoulders. Once in a while these physical reactions to emotions are fine and dandy; in fact they are good—express them! However, say you experience anger every single day; maybe you are in a constant state of rage because of that unbelievably annoying coworker. This continuous tension in your body will begin to cause poor blood circulation and cramping, giving rise to symptoms such as uncomfortable muscle tension, headaches, TMJ, diarrhea and really bad menstrual cramps. Not to mention that chronic anger causes ugly, wrinkly eyebrow furrows!

The way CM sees it is that any emotion experienced excessively (like too much anger or joy) or a failure to fulfill one's desire (whether to quit your job and go back to school or to state what you need in a relationship) makes the Qi of your liver stuck so that it can't properly circulate and do its job. The liver Qi needs to flow smoothly for a body to be nontoxic and in good health. So, each time you have an emotional experience or an unfulfilled desire that you repress or deal with through medication or alcohol, you hamper your liver Qi circulation. Eventually, this chronic repression stagnates your liver Qi so badly that you begin to feel depressed and sad, with little energy to get through your day, let alone the mental clarity to go after what you truly desire. Your poor repressed and unfulfilled body is so jammed up with Qi that it can't digest its food properly, take a healthy poop or circulate blood efficiently and it definitely doesn't feel or look hot, because nothing is moving at the right pace for optimal health. OMG!

Women who take medicine to dull their affect or who repress and ignore their feelings and desires via any other means (even shopping!) are not directly dealing with their emotional states. Whether you ignore pent-up emotions or excessively experience them, they will wreak havoc on your physical body.

Bottom line, ladies: concealing or repressing your emotions and desires will make your liver toxic and you will look and feel unhealthy. You need to feel your emotions, express your emotions, go after your desires and let your liver detox!

By the way, this also works in reverse: living unhealthily will negatively affect your emotional state. Ever notice how you feel depressed, lethargic, bloated and headachy after a night of drinking? This is because your liver is working extra hard to process all the toxic alcohol out of your body. Last night's debauchery has forced your body to put all other tasks aside until it efficiently rids the body of the toxic alcohol overload. This leaves you with the need to lie on the couch all day watching *The Way We Were* and *The English Patient*, crying your eyes out, dehydrated and eating greasy takeout because your body is too toxic and overwhelmed to do anything else. Fun! Ladies, take heed: alcohol is just one example. There are plenty of ways we toxify our bodies on a daily basis: lack of exercise, rage against annoying relatives, not enough sleep, Snickers bars, cigarettes, that third cup of coffee … get my point? These bad habits will render you more prone to an emotional disorder the next time a crisis hits.

I hear you pleading: "Tell me what to do, Aimee!"

In order for your body and mind to remain interconnected, unstuck and sane, girl, you need to

B.E. C.A.L.M.!

- **B**e healthy
- **E**xpress your emotions
- **C**hill the F**k Out
- **A**cknowledge your desires
- **L**et your issues go
- **M**ake it happen

Now, don't go getting overwhelmed on me. These things are very doable. Let me show you.

BE HEALTHY

As I said earlier, the mind is the expression of the body's ability to properly manufacture energy from the foods we eat, how much we sleep and the way we manage our stress. Girls, in order for you to maintain an even emotional keel, you must:

- Eat clean, organic and nondead foods (more on this in the next two chapters).
- Sleep seven to eight hours a night. Period.
- Chill the F**k Out for at least five minutes each day.
- Poop on a regular basis.
- Exercise on a regular basis.

"Being Healthy" pointers can be found throughout the other chapters in this book. Read them and do what I say! Additionally, go ahead and incorporate some of these specific "emotionally balanc-ing" dietary recommendations for depression and anxiety:

Depression

- Eat sour foods like lemons, plums, peaches, raspberries, grapes, olives, apricots, pineapples, mangoes, grapefruit, tangerines and star fruit. In CM theory, the sour taste is said to move liver Qi and cleanse the liver of toxins (emotional and physical) and therefore is great for helping resolve depression.
- Start each day off with a shot of apple-cider vinegar. The vinegar is sour by nature, and as I said above, sour substances move liver Qi and cleanse the liver of toxins (emotional and physical).
- Eat bitter foods like cucumber, dandelion, radish, chive, orange and tangerine peel, fennel, garlic, radish leaf, parsley and spearmint. Bitter foods are particularly good at detoxifying the liver and will help you with your depression.
- Avoid alcohol, caffeine and fatty, greasy, fried foods, as these substances are hard for your liver to process and will further stagnate your depressed liver.

Mary came to see me for depression. She was thirty and had been taking a variety of antidepressant medications over the past eleven years. She had discussed coming off her medication with her therapist and psychiatrist and she wanted me to help.

Chinese Medicine (including acupuncture, Chinese herbs and lifestyle modifications) can really make a profound difference in one's emotional state. By regulating hormones, affecting the release of certain chemicals in your brain and relieving stress, it can make depression less daunting.

When I began working with Mary, she was taking two hundred milligrams of Wellbutrin on a daily basis. Together with her psychiatrist we drew up a plan to slowly wean her off her meds. At my recommendation, she made some dietary changes, began exercising, started taking an individualized Chinese herbal concoction, cut way back on her alcohol intake, began CTFO-ing every day and came for acupuncture once a week. In six months she was off her meds completely. Yes, she still has some rough moments, but I'll never forget when she said to me, "Sure, some days I'm sad—but it's just so good to feel again." When she has a rough day now, she knows she can manage. Her favorite tool is the "Mirror, Mirror" one.

Mary still sees her therapist and has some medication handy if she feels she ever needs it. But all in all she's doing really well.

Anxiety

- Anxiety is viewed in CM theory as a disease that is fiery and hot in nature, so eating foods like oysters, crabs, clams, seaweed, barley, mung beans, lemons, mangoes, oranges, apples, pears, persimmons, watermelons, bananas, grapefruit and star fruit, which are cool in nature, will help chill your anxious soul.
- Eat protein with every meal and snack on nuts, nut butters or hard-boiled eggs. Protein is a natural sedative for the body and will calm your anxiety.
- Drink at least sixty ounces of cool water per day. Water, especially cool or cold water, will help put out the fiery, hot nature of anxiety. Water puts out fire, right?
- Avoid all spicy foods, added sugars and caffeine, as they are naturally hot substances and will heat up your already fiery, hot body and worsen your anxiety.

"EXPRESS YOURSELF" AND STAY HOT LIKE MADONNA

There are many ways you can express yourself beyond dancing in your nipple-tasseled bustier at your favorite nightspot. For more-subtle approaches to expression, find one of the following that works for you and use it, each day; in fact, pick a couple and rotate them. All you have to do is use just ONE of these methods on a daily basis. That's it. It's that easy. The key here is DAILY self-expression. Just adopt one of these habits and begin expressing your emotions, because repression is BAD and it makes your liver toxic and gross and causes you to look older than you are.

- **JOURNALING.** This one is easy. Keep a journal next to your bed and each night before going to sleep, write in it for three to five minutes (remember from chapter three, journaling was part of my recommended daily sixteen-minute regimen). Write about anything that's on your mind. You can make a task list for the next day or a list of errands that need to get done over the weekend, or even write over and over one of the mantras you create for yourself a little later in this chapter. The bottom line is: just write. Express anything that's on your mind. Put it on the paper and get it out of your head! It's liberating!
- **MIRROR, MIRROR.** This one is a little Snow White freakish at first, but you'll see, you can really get into it. Unlike with the journaling, with the "Mirror, Mirror" tool, we're going to say only POSITIVE things. This tool has two parts.

    First, I want you to get used to looking at yourself in the mirror, beyond what it takes to put makeup on. I want you to look into your own eyes and see YOU. Honey, this is harder than you think. Many people have a hard time with this, because the truth is, a lot of people don't like themselves. So first things first, stare deeply into your own eyes and then say sweet, confidence-boosting and loving things like "I love you," "You rock" and "You're the most beautiful woman I've ever met." Do this until you believe yourself. It could take longer than you think. Practice every day. Do this every day for the rest of your life. Girl, women who love themselves are MUCH more beautiful than women who don't.

The second part of the "Mirror, Mirror" tool will have you speaking your own mantra (that you'll create later in this chapter) to your reflection in the mirror every day.

Now, remember, this one is only for POSITIVE talk. If you are in a negative place, put a positive, hopeful spin on things. For example, if what you want to say is "I wish I had a boyfriend," instead say "I allow myself to have a boyfriend"; or if you want to say something like "I am unhappy with the way my career has turned out," instead say "I allow myself to have the career of my dreams." Get it? Just take out the negativity and ALLOW yourself to have what you want. Look in the mirror, love yourself and give yourself permission to have what you desire.

Sometimes I use the "Mirror, Mirror" tool just to have a conversation with myself over something that is on my mind. You can ask yourself questions about the situation and answer yourself in the mirror. It's intriguing to watch the expressions your face makes when you talk about certain situations. Sounds crazy, I know, but don't knock it till you try it!

- **SELF-CENSORING.** No, this doesn't require you tapping your own cell phone. It just requires you to listen to your own internal dialogue. How often do you say mean things to yourself? How often do you berate yourself over things like making a minor mistake at work, or being a klutz or not making your bed or missing your best friend's sister's birthday? Listen to the way you talk to yourself and then ask yourself, "Would I ever talk to my best friend this way?" I hope the answer is NO! Girl, I want you to self-censor and take note of how negative your internal dialogue is. And then, I want you to change it. I want you to say nice, sweet, positive, loving, nondegrading things to yourself. How 'bout the next time you make a mistake, you tell yourself "I love you"? Seriously, it may sound cheesy, but it's better than telling yourself, "you suck." And it'll do wonders for your self-esteem. Give it a shot.

- **TEXT EXPRESS.** This one requires a buddy. Recruit one of your friends to become your Text Express buddy. At some point each day you and your buddy need to *Text Express*: send a text message to each other expressing one emotion you are feeling. It can be as simple as "☺" or "Today is a good day" or as expressive as "Anger. Boss sux. Shitty meetings all morning."

  Maybe it sounds a bit cheesy, but I am telling you—it works! It will help you stay in touch with your emotions and it will give you an outlet to better express yourself. Use it! You'll like it so much you'll eventually want to send more than one message a day.

- **SCREAM.** Pillow necessary (to muffle your screams). This one is for when all you want to do is kick and yell until you feel better. Just grab your pillow and belt it out. It works. It's great for moving out pent-up anger or frustration. Just be sure your neighbors don't call the police.

- **I WANNA PUNCH YOUR LIGHTS OUT.** This may best be done with supervision in a gym. Take a kickboxing class or a regular old boxing lesson or sign up for a martial arts class. Throw some punches. Kick some legs. Let out some grunts. Get out your pent-up bullshit. Kick, punch and grunt your liver toxicity away. It's fun and you're getting a kick-ass workout.

- **BUSTA MOVE.** This is fun and can be done in the privacy of your own home. Just shut the windows, blast your favorite song and dance your butt off. Sing too! You can even throw on your favorite bustier! Dancing feels good, it's good exercise and it's great for getting out some good ol' angst.

  If you're so inclined, take a hip-hop class at your gym or go out and sign yourself up for some dance classes. It's never too late to learn to tango.

- **STOP, DROP AND SIGH.** This can be done anywhere at any time. It's easy. All you have to do is remember to do it. Put a Post-it note on a mirror in your bedroom or your computer screen at work, or set a daily reminder on your phone that says "SDS." And when you are reminded, stop what you're doing, drop your tensed-up shoulders and let out a long and liberating sigh. In CM theory sighing is the sound of the liver, so it is said that when you let out a deep sigh, you are moving stuck liver Qi and therefore helping your liver detox. This is a nice time-out and is great to do when you are feeling particularly stressed. Sigh your stress away.

- **MESSAGE IN A BOTTLE.** This is one of my favorite tools of self-expression: writing a letter or an e-mail that you may never send. Just sit down and write or type a letter to someone you feel you need to express yourself to. Send it if you feel like it or just simply tuck it away on your C drive. Just the act of writing about your emotions, grievances, undying love or lust is therapeutic in and of itself. Unfortunately sometimes the person we feel the need to express ourselves to isn't available; other times it's just not wise to say all the things we may be thinking in the heat of the moment. So write a letter. Say what you need to say. Speak your truth. This even works for people who have passed on. You can still write a letter and say all the things you wish you'd said. It helps. It's cathartic.

- **TELL YOUR STORY.** This may be the most time-consuming self-expression tool, but for some, it really works. Write a short story, start a blog or even write a novel about your life. You can create characters and tell stories; you can share your childhood secrets and vent about your heartbreaks; you can step outside your life and tell your story to a stranger. Creative expression is an amazing tool. Take a writing class, write your story, heal yourself.

CHILL THE F**K OUT

This is your reminder to take your DAILY five-minute CTFO time-out. I go over how to CTFO in chapter 3. Go back and reread it. Do it and make yourself CTFO EVERY DAY!

ACKNOWLEDGE YOUR DESIRES

Over two thousand years ago a great Chinese emperor said that at the root of stagnant liver Qi is one's unfulfilled desires. You see, in CM theory all diseases and illnesses have both a physical and an emotional counterpart; they are often indistinguishable and interdependent. It's like which came first, the chicken or the egg? So if you are walking around with a heart full of unfulfilled desires (and repressed emotions), you can bet your bottom dollar that you are making yourself unhealthy!!

Ladies, let's get to the root of those desires and make them a reality!

First, before we start listing all the things we want and need, let's do a little status report. I want you to get out your pen, look over the four topics I list below and do the following:

- Discuss the current status of the situation.
- Describe the level of fulfillment you receive from the situation.
- Describe your ability or inability to ask for what you need/want from the situation.
- List the first two emotions that come to mind when you think of the situation, choosing from joy/happiness, contentment, anxiety, sorrow, fear, terror, worry or anger/frustration.

1. **WORK**
   a. Current status: What do you do for work? Is it what you want to be doing?
   b. Level of fulfillment: What amount of fulfillment do you receive from your work?
   c. Needs/wants: Do you have the ability to state your needs/wants in the workplace?
   d. Emotional response: What are the first two emotions that come to mind when you think of your work life?

2. **LOVE LIFE**
   a. Current status: What's the current status of your love life?
   b. Level of fulfillment: Are you fulfilled in your love life? If not, then ask yourself why. If yes, ask yourself why (and write the answers here).
   c. Needs/wants: Are you able to ask for what you need/want in a relationship? (Even if you're not in one, do you know what you want/need from a relationship?)
   d. Emotions: What are two emotions that come to mind when you think of your love life?

Kimberly was the self-proclaimed "most anxious, crazy person in Manhattan."

We started working together a couple of months before she was set to move to London with her latest beau. She wanted me to help her become more grounded, sleep better and depend less on Xanax to manage her anxiety.

I remember at her first session she was bouncing off the walls. Most people get really chill after having acupuncture. Not Kimberly. She was bright-eyed and talking a mile a minute after lying down for almost thirty minutes with acupuncture needles in her.

At our next session, I taught her how to breathe. She was a chest breather, meaning she never took a full, deep, fill-your-belly breath. I had her start breathing fifteen real deep belly-rising breaths each night when she got into bed. She started sleeping better. Then she started breathing fifteen real deep belly-rising breaths each morning and she started feeling less anxious.

A month or so later she said to me, in quite an enlightened way, "You know, I think I realized why I was always so anxious—the faster I moved, the less I had to feel the fact that I was so unhappy." Aha!

She started working out what it was she truly wanted out of life. As she learned how to B.E. C.A.L.M., her anxiety left her and she found herself. She still carries her Xanax around with her, just in case she needs it—but those times are few and far between.

3. FRIENDS AND FAMILY
   a. Current status: Do you feel you have a good support system in your friends and family?
   b. Level of fulfillment: Do you get fulfillment from relationships with friends and family, or do they feel one-sided and draining? Or maybe both? Discuss.
   c. Needs/wants: Are you able to ask for what you need/want in your relationships with your friends and family?
   d. Emotions: What are the first two emotions that come to mind when you think of (1) your friends, (2) your family?

4. HEALTH
   a. Current status: Do you feel you are in good health? Are you taking any medications to manage a health-care issue? If so, how do you feel about taking the prescribed medication?
   b. Level of fulfillment: Does your state of health allow you to go after your desires?
   c. Needs/wants: Do you have the resources/support system to maintain or improve your state of health? Do you use these resources?
   d. Emotions: What are the first two emotions that come to mind when you think of your health? If you take medications to manage your health, what are the first two emotions that come to mind when you think of those medicines?

Read over your answers to the above questions and then I want you to ask yourself:

How fulfilled am I in my life?

Girl, this is the million-dollar question. It's not meant to depress you—it is meant only to bring you perspective on your current state of fulfillment. Sit with this question for a while. In fact, take a CTFO break right now and ponder this question. Five minutes, give 'em to me right now.

What is the answer you came up with? Are you as fulfilled as you want to be in your life, or are certain situations holding you back?

With your above self-survey and level of fulfillment in mind, I want you to list one desire you wish to fulfill THIS YEAR that correlates with each of the four topics above. This desire should be something tangible that you think would make your life, right now, more fulfilling. It cannot be that new Jimmy Choo espadrille or a new car. We are talking about emotional fulfillment relating to the four topics you've just surveyed. Is it a new job, or more responsibility at your job? Is it a more-fulfilling love life or a deeper friendship with your mother? Is it to stop taking a certain medication or to better manage your health? Really think about these desires and give this your all. Your health and happiness are hinging on it!

To help you out a bit, here are my desires:

1. **WORK:** the ability to delegate my office workload efficiently while I am writing this book
2. **LOVE LIFE:** to allow myself a healthy romantic relationship (that leads to marriage) where I have the ability to ask for what I need and maintain my independence
3. **FRIENDS/FAMILY:** to dedicate more time to building a relationship with my brother
4. **HEALTH:** to make time for a daily twenty-minute meditation

All right, now it's your turn:

1. **WORK:**

2. **LOVE LIFE:**

3. **FRIENDS/FAMILY:**

4. Health:

OK, now that we have some clear-cut desires to go after, we are going to move on to letting go of the emotions that are holding us back from our desires, and then we are going to make those desires happen!

LET IT GO

Before we get to the "making our desires happen" section, we must first learn to let go of what is holding us back. This is the fun stuff! Before we can fulfill ourselves, we need to learn to let go of our patterns of self-loathing and self-deprecation that ultimately prevent us from going after our deepest desires. Get ready, girl: this is where we get to the bottom of what you still beat yourself up over and what you don't allow yourself to have because of repressed need-to-let-go-of emotions.

I want you to look at your four desires above and I want you to take two minutes and fantasize about each of these desires individually, asking yourself what having these desires fulfilled would look and feel like. What would it feel like to have the perfect job? What would it look like to be in love with your soul mate? What would it feel like to have optimal health? As you run through each of these fantasies, I want you to see if you're afraid of anything surrounding the fantasy. Are you scared that having the perfect job would change the relationship you have with your close friends? Are you scared that having your one true love in your life would rob you of your independence? Get the idea?

Along with taking note of what scary and fearful emotions came up surrounding your fantasies, I want you to take each of your four desires and list which emotion or emotions you feel are keeping you from desire "X" (joy, worry, fear, anxiety, sorrow/sadness, terror, anger). Chances are it's one or both of the emotions you attached to the topic in the above section.

For example, here are the emotions I feel are keeping me from fulfilling my four desires:

1. **WORK:** anxiety and worry over my ability to allow someone else to help run my business
2. **LOVE LIFE:** fear of vulnerability, fear of losing my independence as I have in the past
3. **FAMILY/FRIENDSHIPS:** sorrow for the emotional rifts that still exist
4. **HEALTH:** anxiety over time management

Your turn. Write the emotion that you feel may be holding you back from your top four desires here:

1. Emotion preventing "work desire":
2. Emotion preventing "love-life desire":
3. Emotion preventing "friendship/family desire":
4. Emotion preventing "health desire":

All right, ladies, we are about to create your new mantras so that you can learn to LET GO of the emotions that are holding you back. I want you to take each emotion and desire you wrote above and plug them into the sentence below:

"I allow myself to let go of x **[**x **= whatever emotion you listed] and I allow myself to** y **[**y **= the desire you want fulfilled]."**

For example: *I allow myself to let go of fear and I allow myself a healthy romantic relationship (that leads to marriage) where I can maintain my independence and ask for what I need.*

Write your new mantras here:

1. **WORK:** I allow myself to let go of _____ and I allow myself _____
   _____
   _____
   _____

2. **LOVE LIFE:** I allow myself to let go of _____ and I allow myself _____

_____

_____

_____

3. **FAMILY/FRIENDSHIPS:** I allow myself to let go of _____ _____ and I allow myself

_____

_____

_____

4. **HEALTH:** I allow myself to let go of _____ and I allow myself _____

_____

_____

_____

This is where the "Mirror, Mirror" tool comes into play: I want you to say each mantra out loud into your bathroom mirror. When you do this, do yourself a favor and say it like you mean it. Own that mantra. Don't be a wimp! Let go of the emotions that are holding you back from your desires!

Say your first mantra ten times DAILY into your mirror-mirror-on-the-wall and then move on to the next mantra the following week. Take your time with this. Your goal is to focus on one mantra per week and then move on to the next one on the list until all four are done. After the four weeks are up, repeat the cycle.

Now, don't get freaked—remembering to do this is easy. Just get out a Post-it, write all four mantras on it and tape it to your mirror. (If you're nervous about what others may think if they see your Post-it, make this your first week's mantra: "I allow myself to let go of fear and anxiety of what others think of me and I allow myself thriving mental health.") As you finish each week, check off the mantra you've completed and move on to the next one.

When you fulfill one of the listed desires, or you've uncovered something new worth letting go of, come up with a new mantra and add it to the list.

Remember: say each sentence like you mean it. Own it. Let the emotions go and get what you desire!

Extra Credit

If you want to go another step deeper into the lovely self-deprecation black hole, think about something that happened that you still haven't forgiven yourself for. What are the first memories that come to mind? I want you to remember the moment; try to relive it in your head; spend some time with it. Whom were you with? Do you have any regrets? If so, what are they? What would you have done differently? Run through the memory, taking notes if necessary. Next, I want you to say out loud fifteen times while you look into your own eyes in the mirror, "I did the best I could. I forgive myself for _____. I can let this go."

Forgiving yourself and saying it out loud can be done with just about anything. I want you to use this tool as much as you need to. I want you to learn to let things go. The past is the past and it can't be changed. All we can do is direct our energy each day in a positive manner so that we allow ourselves to be fulfilled today. Now! Do it! Girl, forgive yourself. You deserve it!

MAKE IT HAPPEN

Now that you have identified and are letting go of the emotions that are holding you back from fulfilling your desires, you are one step closer to making your desires your reality. Here is where we learn to Make It Happen.

Girl, in order for you to make your desires a reality, you must envision them. This is going to require you to really, serious-as-a-heart-attack do your daily five-minute CTFO times.

What would it look like if you loved your job? Or if you had perfect health?

Let's imagine it.

Get out your pencils again. And in each of the designated areas I want you to write out what your fulfilled desires would look like and feel like. I want you to imagine them, feel them, smell them. What would you wear? How would your life be?

OK, let's try this out. Next to each of your four desires I want you to write one sentence using a descriptive adjective to express how you would feel once you allowed yourself to have it.

For example, if we were talking about the work desire, you might say something like, "I would feel liberated if I was able to ask for help preparing for the Monday morning meeting."

Now take that descriptive adjective and imagine what it would feel like. What would being liberated feel like? Would your shoulders drop? Would your headache go away? Would your daily work rage be tamed? Think about it—envision feeling liberated at work!! CTFO on it.

Get your pencils ready. . . .

1. **WORK:** I would feel _____ if I allowed myself to have _____
   _____

2. **LOVE LIFE:** I would feel _____ if I allowed myself to have_____
   _____

3. **FAMILY/FRIENDSHIP:** I would feel _____ if I allowed myself to have _____
   _____

4. **HEALTH:** I would feel _____ if I allowed myself to have _____
   _____

When you're feeling defeated—repeat these sentences to yourself and feel that good feeling, be that adjective, make it happen.

Getting closer to your desires is your choice and you can do it. You just have to peel through the layers of junk you've tucked away over the years. Let go of fear and dive into life. It is yours for the taking.

If you want to meet a man, own it. Don't be afraid to do the on-line thing. Don't be afraid to ask your friends to set you up. Imagine it and allow yourself to have it.

Tell me, what would your ideal relationship *realistically* look like? What would the ultimate job be for you? How would it make you feel? Feel that feeling, hold on to it and make it real. We can't get to where we want to be if we don't know what we truly want. Girl, figure out what you truly desire and how it would feel if it was yours, and make it happen!

All right, ladies, now you know how to fight the perils of aging by prioritizing your happiness and peace, deprioritizing your stress and CTFO-ing on a daily basis, and how to B.E. C.A.L.M. and battle the evils of anxiety and depression. Next, I'm going to show you how to seriously amp up your health by avoiding what I call the Big Four phlegm-producing foods. Read on, we're only gettin' started! Optimal health is at your fingertips. Make it happen!

5.

sugar is evil.
soy sucks.
Bigger is not Better.

𝒥 WAS IN the Barneys fitting room one Saturday afternoon, trying on an overpriced pair of "skinny" jeans. In the fitting room next to me, two women were talking:

"Should I get them?" one woman asked.

"They're hot!" her friend replied.

"But does my ass look like a shelf?"

"A shelf?" her friend asked, laughing.

"I swear, I've been starving myself for these jeans!"

Both girls broke into hysterics as I began surveying my own ass, wondering if it, in fact, looked like a shelf.

"All I had for lunch today was that bag of M&M's," Ms. Shelf-Ass said.

"That's more than I've eaten all day!" the other countered.

My heart dropped and my face went red with anger.

When are women going to grow out of the idea that starving themselves is a good thing? When are women going to realize that a bag of M&M's offers them absolutely zilch for nourishment?

M&M's are just like that flaky guy you dumped three years ago who still calls you at three a.m. on Fridays. They are both LOSERS that will never address your needs and will cause more harm than good.

Let's look at the ingredients in a bag of M&M's: sugar, chocolate, milk, cocoa butter, lactose, soy lecithin, salt, cornstarch, corn syrup, gum acacia, Red 40 Lake, Blue 2 Lake, Yellow 5, Yellow 6, Blue 1 Lake, Red 40, Blue 1, dextrin.

Beyond the sugar, chocolate, milk and salt, can you tell me where the other ingredients come from? Do you know where you can find a soy lecithin tree or a Blue 2 Lake?

Maybe in Alice's Wonderland? No, probably not even there.

Let me break it down for you:

- Cocoa butter is vegetable fat mechanically derived from cocoa beans.
- Lactose is another name for a processed dairy sugar.
- Soy lecithin is chemically extracted soybean-oil fat, which the FDA has stated is "virtually" nontoxic, i.e., sketchy at best.
- Cornstarch is starch derived from corn.
- Corn syrup is another type of processed sugar.
- Gum acacia is another type of processed sugar.
- Red, Blue and Yellow are all chemically processed food dyes that are "virtually" nontoxic ... sketchy!
- Dextrin is yet another name for processed sugar.

So, M&M's are basically processed sugar, "virtually" nontoxic additives and colorings and a wee bit of nonorganic, hormone- and antibiotic-filled cow's milk, nonorganic chocolate and salt. Does this sound nutritious to you? I think you're smarter than that, and you know that M&M's are not food! Right?

Food occurs naturally, in nature. Food grows on trees and in the dirt, comes from the sea or walks on legs. Food is not born in a laboratory in New Jersey.

The purpose of food is to provide our bodies fuel to function. In

Chinese Medicine theory, proper nourishment—food that contributes to our daily energy, overall state of health and longevity—comes from eating naturally occurring, fresh foods: foods that are as close to their natural state as possible (like an organic apple or broccoli stalk).

Nourishment does NOT come from Blue 2 Lake or soy lecithin and it definitely doesn't come from starvation! You should not be eating processed foods that are chemically engineered, synthetically derived or artificially flavored.

In CM, we view processed foods as dead. D-E-A-D. This is because processed foods are artificial and contain chemicals that our bodies can neither recognize nor use as nutrients. Processed foods contain preservatives that allow them to sit at the bottom of your purse for an eternity and never, ever go bad. Once inside your body, these never-go-bad, dead, processed foods sit in your digestive system as indigestible matter that causes toxic cellular debris to build up—and voilà, you now have a shelflike cellulite-filled ass. Oh no!

Here's a mantra you need to live by:

If it sits on your counter (or in the bottom of your purse) and it doesn't go bad—DON'T EAT IT.

Bottom line: if you consume alive—nondead—and nutrient-rich ingredients that are naturally occurring, you will in time become a healthier person. If you consume processed and chemically manufactured dead ingredients that your body cannot digest, you will increase your chances of one day being diagnosed with a chronic disease like cancer, diabetes, osteoporosis, depression or heart disease. It's a simple fact; this is NOT an opinion.

Girls, this means you need to eat alive—nondead—foods. Not dead "meal replacement" bars. You need to eat foods that are naturally rich in nutrients and fat and vitamins and minerals. Not a container of "healthy" fat-free, sugar-free, chemical-laden frozen yogurt. You need to eat foods that your body can digest so that it can function and be healthy. Not indigestible foods like soy (see the

"Soy Sucks" section in this chapter for more juice on the perils of soy).

Before I tell you what foods you need to ditch like a lame boyfriend (chapter 6 will tell you what foods you *should* be eating), let me first explain the digestive process.

CM theory teaches that the process of digestion involves the spleen and the stomach. In CM, not only does the spleen carry out its physiological processes as understood in Western terms, but it also works in conjunction with the stomach to warm the food and drink that enters the body, digest it, separate it into its "pure" and "impure" parts and disperse it throughout the body. The "pure" stuff is saved and becomes the body's energy to function optimally and the "impure" stuff is recognized for what it is, waste, and it is excreted into places such as your toilet bowl, your liver, the cellulite on your thighs and the pimples on your back! Ewww!

At the end of the day the "pure" stuff that hasn't been used up by the body to function is transformed into what we call postnatal essence.

"Huh? Postnatal essence? Is that the stuff that makes my hair shinier?"

Essence is not a hair product. If you remember, we talked about essence in chapter 3: it's the foundation of our health and longevity and it is stored in our body (specifically our kidneys) as an energetic reserve. And do you remember how in chapter 3 I said you could actually make more essence? Well, now I'm going to explain how. But first let me explain about the two types of essence:

- Prenatal essence is before-birth essence, the foundation from which we are created. This includes not only what some would refer to as our genetics but also the embryonic environment in which we developed. So if Mom was a smoker who ate mainly processed foods and hated her job, we didn't get the best prenatal essence. Conversely if she was the happiest, healthiest pregger, we had a great embryonic environment and received a nice chunk of prenatal essence. Unfortunately, prenatal essence is completely out of our control.

- Postnatal essence is after-birth essence. This is the health and longevity that we can create by eating and living as naturally as possible. This is the stuff you can build all on your own. Girl, the ball is in your court. Postnatal essence is critical and can override a negative embryonic environment or a bad dose of prenatal essence and have a positive effect on our genetic predispositions!

"Really, how I live my life can affect my genetic predispositions?" you ask.

Yes!

Even if you weren't reared in an optimal embryonic environment or bequeathed an ideal genetic makeup, you can compensate for those disadvantages (say, a predisposition to breast cancer or high cholesterol) and improve your current and long-term health by eating clean and living peacefully. In fact, Western science is finally catching up with Chinese Medicine's two-thousand-year-old theory of postnatal essence. Many scientists are researching environmental cues (or, as they are known in the scientific community, "epigenetic factors") such as diet and tobacco smoke and their positive or negative impact on one's genetic predisposition and the development of certain diseases such as cancer. In fact, researchers at the University of Alabama at Birmingham recently published a report in *The American Journal of Human Genetics* that identical twins, with very similar genes, can display different physical manifestations depending on the environmental cues, or epigenetic factors, they are exposed to. John Witte, a professor of genetic epidemiology at the University of California, San Francisco, stated in the *New York Times*, regarding epigenetic-factor research, "You've got a little bit more genetic variation than previously thought."

Bottom line: the more of this postnatal essence we rack up, the healthier we will be, the longer we will live, the fewer diseases we will be predisposed to and the better our skin will look.

Ladies, postnatal essence is all the rage.

But we can't give our bodies the energy to create any postnatal essence if all we eat is impure, dead and chemically treated food. Impure foods don't jibe with our digestive system.

What happened the last time you ate a Luna bar or soft-serve frozen yogurt? I betcha you got tired, had gas and felt bloated. If you're a sensitive Sally like myself, your eczema may even have flared up!

Impure and overly processed foods impair your digestion, make your insides sticky and, as we like to say in CM, create phlegm. Yes, phlegm! Like the green stuff you cough up or blow out your nose. As we all know, phlegm is thick, dense and heavy; it's gross. When this goopy phlegm accumulates in your digestive system from all the impure foods you ingest, the spleen and stomach get confused and they can no longer decipher pure foods from impure ones. Now you are left with an inefficient digestive system that is phlegm filled and too weak to create postnatal essence, not to mention a poor metabolism and the potential to develop all sorts of diseases such as hypothyroidism, diabetes, heart disease, cancer and infertility.

Look around for phlegmy people. They are prone to crappy skin with pimples (think of the viscous, phlegmlike substance known as sebum that comes out of a zit), cellulite, dry and brittle hair, thyroid disorders, diabetes, infertility, pooping problems, extra fat in places they don't want it and bags under their eyes.

Open your eyes. Dead-processed-food-eating people are everywhere!

Every time you eat an impure food and experience gas, bloating or maybe even urgent diarrhea, I'd like you to imagine a big ball of phlegm sitting in your stomach.

And, just to scare you a little bit more, phlegm, when accumulated over long periods of time, gums up the entire body and severely retards the flow of Qi and blood and becomes things like excess cholesterol, cysts (like ovarian, uterine or breast), polyps (like the ones that can pop up in your colon), fatty deposits (like the ones that often occur on the liver) and tumors. In CM, phlegm is considered the main contributor in the development of cancer.

Yes, cancer!

But don't freak. In order for you to get back to health and to maintain your health, you just need to stop eating processed phlegm-creating foods!

The Big Four phlegm-producing foods that we need to steer clear of are

- sugar
- soy
- white flour
- dairy (except in moderation—I'll tell how much and why a bit later in this chapter).

Remembering these Big Four phlegm-producing foods is quite easy. Just memorize the following mantra:

Don't Eat Anything White.

This is the moment when you should start rethinking that Starbucks white-flour-based morning pastry and white-sugar-filled white soy semidry mocha latte.

All right, now let's discuss each of the Big Four individually.

· SUGAR IS EVIL AND IT DOESN'T GIVE · A HOOT ABOUT YOUR POSTNATAL ESSENCE

Girls, sugar is one of the biggest evils of ALL time!

When I'm talking about sugar, I am not talking about the sugars in fruits and vegetables; those are the "good" sugars—great sugars, in fact—that actually offer our body wholesome nutrients and naturally occurring vitamins.

When I speak of sugar, I am talking specifically about "added sugars": things like high-fructose corn syrup, crystalline fructose, table sugar, cane sugar, sucrose and corn syrup (see the box on the next page for the common names of added sugars).

Chances are, you are ingesting a lot more sugar than you actually know.

Sugar in Disguise!

Other common names for added sugar:

beet sugar	high-fructose corn syrup
brown sugar	lactose
cane syrup or juice	malt syrup (rice, barley)
confectioners' sugar	maltodextrin
corn syrup	maltose
crystalline fructose	maple sugar
dextrin	molasses
dextrose	Sucanat
evaporated cane juice	sucrose
fructose	turbinado
galactose	xylose
glucose	

I had a patient come in for her first visit drinking a bottle of Vitaminwater. After some introductory questions, I asked her if her diet consisted of a lot of sugar.

"No, not really," she said. "I don't drink soda anymore and I have the occasional dessert, but I really try to avoid sugar."

I asked her to take a look at the label on her Vitaminwater and tell me how many grams of sugar it had.

"Thirteen grams per serving. Is that bad?"

Uh … yeah! First of all, I encourage patients to avoid more than ten grams of added sugar per day. Second of all, a "serving" is defined on that bottle as eight ounces, meaning there are actually two and a half servings in that twenty-ounce bottle and a whopping total of 32.5 grams of sugar! That's eight teaspoons of sugar—a twelve-ounce can of soda contains nine teaspoons of sugar. That's a slim difference between Vitaminwater and a can of soda.

"The marketing made me do it. It has 'vitamin' in the name!" she protested. "So, you're saying this is bad for me? What about all the vitamins?"

I have to agree, the marketing is very misleading. Not only is that drink unhealthy, but the so-called vitamins it contains are completely synthetic and almost entirely unabsorbable by your body. And its sugar content will completely overwhelm your digestive system, preventing you from receiving nutrients from any "pure" foods you may decide to eat the rest of the day.

In CM, sugar is the biggest evil phlegm substance out there. It will hamper digestion and make your insides murky and gross, cause an overgrowth of bacteria in your colon, make you feel foggy-headed and fatigued, cause conditions like high cholesterol and acid reflux and make your outsides blemished and brimming with flab and cellulite!

Here's why: refined, concentrated sweeteners like high-fructose corn syrup and crystalline fructose overwhelm the spleen and stomach, causing them to generate large amounts of phlegmy fluid in the body. This phlegmy fluid offers the body nothing for nourishment and all your physiological functions will suffer and slow down.

Word to the wise: added sugars are in EVERYTHING and Americans are eating it by the bucketful. According to U.S. Department of Agriculture (USDA) data, sugar consumption in 1999 was 158 pounds per person—thirty percent higher than what it was in 1983. Think about that: 158 pounds of sugar per person every year, or put another way, the average American ingests FIFTY TEASPOONS of "added sugar" per day! OMG!

The official U.S. guidelines advise a maximum of forty grams (that's ten teaspoons per day!) of refined sugar for every two thousand calories consumed. Unfortunately, this "guideline" is one of the reasons, according to the *Journal of the American Heart Association*, that the incidence of type 2 diabetes among middle-aged Americans has doubled over the last three decades.

And get this: high-fructose corn syrup and crystalline fructose, the two biggest added sugars used by the food industry, both contain arsenic. Yup, you heard me, freaking arsenic. The stuff that is used to poison insects and varmints! And it doesn't just stop at arsenic. Both crystalline fructose and high-fructose corn syrup also contain lead, chloride and other noxious heavy metals. Mmmmmm … soooo good!!

Ladies, added sugars are EVIL, they are in EVERYTHING and they are giving you bad skin, gastrointestinal disorders and type 2 diabetes and poisoning you.

Read your labels. Steer clear of processed added sugars. They are poisonous, pervasive and predisposing you to a plethora of illnesses.

Word to the Wise:
Artificial Sweeteners Are Not So Sweet!

Bottom line: these things are chemicals and they are toxic. Don't ingest them! Scientists have found that Aspartame, aka Nutra-Sweet, lowers serotonin levels, exacerbating disorders like depression, headaches, migraines and seizures.

Try cutting out that daily diet soda and see if your afternoon headache doesn't go away.

Common names for artificial sweeteners:

Aspartame Cyclamate Maltitol Mannitol Saccharin Sorbitol Xylitol Sunette NutraSweet Equal

---

• SOY SUCKS •

Don't eat soy. Let me say it again: don't eat soy products. Surprised? Let me tell you why.

Soy products on the whole are processed and toxic. Eating soy may make your period irregular and compromise your ability to get pregnant; it can give you osteoporosis, horrible gas, zero energy and hypothyroidism (and I'll tell you why in just a sec ...). It's also one of the most common food allergens. I am not joking. Do not eat it!

The vegan-preaching soy supporters out there have neglected to tell the general population that most soy products on the market are made from overly processed and more than likely genetically modified soybeans that have the nutritional equivalent of plastic. In fact, in the 1930s, the late, great Henry Ford invested over a million dollars in soy research for its potential industrial use. So what did this research discover? That soybean oil made a superior enamel for painting automobiles and that it was a great plastic alternative. Ford loved the cheap crop so much he used it not only in car paint but also in horn buttons, gearshift knobs, door handles, window trim, accelerator pedals and timing gears in every Ford car. You see, the high temperatures at which your favorite "faux duck" and "fakin' bacon" are processed cause all sorts of proteins to denature (i.e., to break apart and lose the enzymatic activity that allows us to digest them). This high-temperature processing renders the food virtually inedible. But it makes a great paint enamel and plastic substitute!

"But what about all the healthy Asian people who have been eating it for thousands of years?"

People in Asian countries have not been eating "nofurkey" or "sham ham" for the last three thousand years. Traditionally, Asians consumed nonprocessed, non-genetically modified (GM), fermented soy, also known as miso—and they ate this fermented soy as a side dish, not a main course (that's not to say that with the Americanization of Asia hasn't come the introduction of more processed and nonfermented soy products).

FYI: I'd bet my thumbs on the fact that the tofu or any soy-based product you're eating—regardless if it's non-GM, organic or "all natural"—is overly processed, loaded with additives and carcinogens and NOT fermented.

Are you confused yet?

Let's break down these two differences.

First: The soy products you eat are processed. The act of processing soy requires very high temperatures, which denatures important enzymes that our body needs to digest soy. As well, processing soy creates toxins and carcinogens like nitrates and MSG that are so unhealthy for us it's appalling.

Second: The soy products you eat are NOT fermented. The process of fermentation "predigests" soy, allowing it to be easily absorbed. Fermentation also neutralizes the natural toxins found in soy. All fermented foods are also rich in probiotics, which introduce friendly bacteria into our digestive tract. The probiotic activity in fermented foods such as miso is great for boosting the immune system, improving digestive health and fighting off the damage done by too many phlegmy foods! So, you can see how fermented soy may actually be good for one's health.

Just to reiterate: we are eating processed and nonfermented soy products. Traditional Asian diets consisted of soy products that were NOT processed and were fermented.

Get the difference?

Here's another difference. Several scientific studies published by established journals like *The Journal of Nutrition, Nutrition and Cancer* and *Nutrition Research* have found that the daily soy FOOD consumption throughout Asia ranges between two and forty-eight grams of soy FOOD per day. **Let me be clear: that's grams of soy FOOD per day, not grams of soy PROTEIN per day.**

"Huh?"

You see, the typical American vegetarian, vegan, pseudo-vegetarian or straight up carnivore who believes soy is healthy can easily ingest one cup of tofu or one glass of soy milk on a daily basis ... and sometimes both! One cup (or eight ounces) of tofu or one glass (or eight ounces) of soy milk is roughly equivalent to 224 grams of soy FOOD. In looking at the numbers—the average Asian ingests twenty-five grams of soy FOOD per day, and the average American can ingest 224 grams—there's a whopping difference. Basically, Americans who are eating soy products daily consume almost ten times more grams of soy FOOD (or about seven times more ounces) per day than what is found in the typical Asian diet.

And when it comes to soy PROTEIN, the typical soy-is-healthy-for-me American is ingesting anywhere from ten to forty grams per day, whereas the typical Asian person, following a traditional diet, ingests one to seven grams of soy PROTEIN per day.

Big difference.

So you can figure out how much soy PROTEIN you were eating before you read this section and decided to NEVER eat soy again:

- Four ounces of tofu contains twelve grams of soy PROTEIN.
- One soy "sausage" link contains six grams of soy PROTEIN.
- One soy "burger" contains ten to thirteen grams of soy PROTEIN.
- An eight-ounce glass of plain soy milk contains seven grams of soy PROTEIN.
- One soy protein bar contains fourteen grams of soy PROTEIN.
- One-half cup of tempeh contains nineteen and a half grams of soy PROTEIN.
- A quarter cup of soy nuts contains twenty-four grams of soy PROTEIN.

Here's a good measuring tool: each ounce of soy FOOD contains approximately three grams of soy PROTEIN.

Keep in mind, one ounce = twenty-eight grams.

Bottom line: the amount of soy PROTEIN in the traditional Asian diet is much less than what's in the current American soy-is-the-panacea diet. And, Asians are typically consuming a completely different nonprocessed, fermented soy product.

"But what about the phytoestrogens in soy that I've heard so much about? Don't they help fight off breast cancer?"

Phytoestrogens are plant estrogens that are very similar to our own body's estrogen, only weaker.

Sue came to see me because she wanted to lose weight. She heard acupuncture could help boost her metabolism. As we talked, I learned that she had been a vegetarian (although she still ate fish) for the last ten years. . . . You know where this is going, don't you?

Basically she was eating butt loads of soy! She had no energy, a completely irregular I-bleed-so-heavy-I-can't-leave-the-house menstrual cycle. She also had fibrocystic breasts that were "constantly" killing her. But the most frustrating thing of all was that even with zilch for energy she was exercising five days a week and she still couldn't lose weight.

Well, I told her, just as I am telling you—soy ain't so sexy. In fact, it sucks. She didn't believe me, so I flat out begged her to give up soy (and I inundated her with scientific research displaying the perils of soy).

She did it.

A year later, she eats meat and not soy. And her period's regular, her boobs don't hurt, she has energy, she exercises AND she's lost fifteen pounds!

So, one scientific theory holds that the weaker plant estrogen in soy will replace the stronger body estrogen, making you less estrogenic and less likely to develop estrogen-dependent diseases such as breast, ovarian and uterine cancer.

Sure, that sounds good. In theory. In reality, soy is not so sexy and over time actually makes you more estrogenic and more likely to get estrogen-dependent diseases! Over the last decade, several groups of scientists published articles in journals like *Cancer Research, The Journal of Nutrition* and *Carcinogenesis* displaying evidence that the phytoestrogen components in soy stimulate the growth of breast cancer cells and cause abnormal cell growth (which is an indicator of cancer) in reproductive tissues of female rodents. One group of researchers even found that the more processed the soy product was, the faster it caused cancer to grow! Some would argue about the relevance of these studies, as they were carried out on rodents and not humans, but—the evidence is confounding enough for me to tell you to never eat soy again, especially nonfermented, processed and genetically modified soy.

Let me explain why: processed soy foods, like the ones sold throughout most of America, are essentially indigestible, especially genetically modified ones. So what actually happens is, over time, these plant estrogens from soy, although weaker, wind up accumulating in your body and actually increase your chances of developing the bad estrogen-dominant diseases like ovarian cancer, endometriosis, uterine fibroids, infertility and breast cancer. Not to mention that women with too much estrogen tend to have too much weight around their abdomens, raging PMS and depression. You see, over the short term, these plant estrogens seem good, but after a period of time (say one month of daily ingestion of tofu, "nofurkey" or a health food store–bought soy supplement) these excess plant estrogens create a toxic, estrogenic and cancerous environment inside your body!

"But, Aimee, I rarely eat soy products!"

Think again. Even if you don't drink soy milk or have a hankering for tofu, you are consuming soy. It is estimated that sixty percent of packaged and processed foods (even the ones in health-food stores) contain soy in the form of soy protein isolate, soy lecithin, soy oil and soy flour. It's soy mania out there. Soy protein isolate (SPI) is probably the worst culprit of them all. This SPI junk is made from defatted soybean flakes that have been washed in either alcohol or water to remove sugars and dietary fiber. Yummy! Can I have some more defatted soy flakes!

Ladies, it's not enough to stop eating your prized tofu dishes and soy milk. You also have to start reading labels because soy protein isolate and a slew of other processed soy products are in EVERYTHING. Lucky us, we can find these processed soy derivatives (see box) in "health" bars, protein shakes, tomato sauce, Mountain Dew, bottled fruit drinks, soups, breads, ice cream, baked goods and breakfast cereals.

These noxious, processed soy derivatives popped up everywhere back in 1999 when the FDA decided that it was a health benefit for adults to eat twenty-five grams of soy protein per day (FYI: that's the equivalent of eight ounces of tofu or one soy protein bar).

Just to be clear, the FDA's recommended twenty-five grams of soy protein per day is four times more soy protein than the one to seven grams consumed per day in traditional Asian diets—not to mention that the traditional Asian diets consisted of nonprocessed and fermented soy, NOT defatted soy flakes.

"Aimee, how could this have happened?!"

You got me.

In 1991, Japanese researchers reported that consumption of as little as thirty grams or two tablespoons of soybeans per day for only one month resulted in a significant increase in thyroid-stimulating hormone, causing hypothyroidism and goiter. The *American Journal of Clinical Nutrition* published a study in 1994 that showed that after women ate sixty grams of soy protein (not food) per day for thirty days, their menstrual cycle changed, resulting in skipped ovulations and irregular menstruation for three months following the cessation of eating soy protein! In 1998 the same journal published another study stating that ingestion of sixty grams per day of soy protein for fourteen days caused fibrocystic breast changes (a potential precursor to breast cancer) in American women. In 2007 the

Journal of Medicinal Food posted a study that found that phytoestrogen intake in adult female rats affected their uterine linings, making them hyperplastic. This means that dietary plant estrogens make the uterine lining thicker, uneven, less fertile and more likely to develop fibroids or cancer. YUCK!

Get this: toxicologist Michael Fitzpatrick, Ph.D., found that a way to induce thyroid cancer in laboratory animals was to give them thyroid-boosting drugs such as Synthroid while also feeding them thyroid-inhibiting foods such as soy. If you have thyroid issues, I hope your endocrinologist made you aware of the dangers of soy before prescribing your Synthroid. If not, go talk to her about your diet and your meds.

Guess what? Soy is bad for babies too. In 2008, the *Journal of Pediatric Gastroenterology and Nutrition* published an article stating that female infants fed soy-based formulas were developing breast buds by the age of two! Babies fed soy-based formula have thirteen thousand to twenty-two thousand times more estrogen compounds in their blood than babies fed milk-based formula.

Ladies, I want you to read this sentence twice:

Infants exclusively fed soy formula receive the estrogenic equivalent of at least five birth control pills per day.

Holy shit!

Guess what? Soy is bad for men too. Dr. Jorge Chavarro, a researcher from Harvard, recently presented to the American Society for Reproductive Medicine results from clinical studies investigating the effects of soy-derived foods on human sperm quality. What did his research conclude? The consumption of soy foods is linked to lower sperm concentration. Yup! Girl, if you want babies, get your boy off soy!

So what about the scientific studies the soy industry and the FDA quote to tout the benefits of soy? Well, most of them, like the one published in 1997 by *Clinical and Investigative Medicine*, lasted an average of only four weeks. So maybe they didn't run their studies long enough to realize the deleterious effects of soy? What's also interesting is that these "benefits of soy" media claims report only the potential positives, such as lower LDL cholesterol and decreased breast cancer risk (by the way, the American Heart Association recently revised its stance on these claims—details are below). But if you go back and look at these actual soy studies, you'll see that what's left out is not only the short duration of the study but also that most of the subjects who ingested twenty-five grams per day of soy had foul farts, diarrhea, rashes and vomiting. Oh, Soy Not Sexy!

"But, Aimee, the studies you quoted to knock soy ran for only four weeks too."

Nope. The studies I quoted ran for longer than four weeks, but it was at the four-week point that researchers began to notice the NEGATIVE effects of soy. Prior to this four-week threshold, soy was seemingly beneficial to the subjects. So the point I am trying to make is, the studies used to promote the "health benefits" of soy did not run long enough to show the harmful side effects of soy. Make sense?

If you're still not convinced, here's the clincher: in 2006 the American Heart Association published the *Soy Protein, Isoflavones and Cardiovascular Health* science advisory after reviewing all of the scientific research that had been conducted on the health benefits of soy from 1996 to 2006; their conclusion: "Thus, the direct cardiovascular health benefit of soy protein or isoflavone supplements is minimal at best. Soy protein or isoflavones have not been shown to improve vasomotor symptoms of menopause, and results are mixed with regard to the slowing of postmenopausal bone loss. The efficacy and safety of soy isoflavones for preventing or treating cancer of the breast, endometrium, and prostate are not established; evidence from clinical trials is meager and cautionary with regard to a possible adverse effect. For this reason, use of (soy) isoflavone supplements in food or pills is not recommended."

Did you catch the part about a possible adverse effect?

Wow.

• • •

Well, as I've stressed already in this book, everything in moderation. But if you don't need to eat it, don't.

We know that genetically modified (GM) soy and any processed soy derivatives (like soy protein isolate, soy lecithin, textured vegetable protein, soy oil and soy flour) offer us zilch for nutrition and are BAD for us, so don't eat them. If you absolutely need to have something with soy in it, be sure it is NON-GM and fermented, and have no more than one two-ounce serving (about six grams of soy protein) two times per week.

Who knows what health woes will arise in those who eat the FDA-recommended twenty-five grams of soy protein per day for several years? Thyroid explosion? A second uterus? Man boobs?

Here are some more bad, bad things about processed, nonfermented soy eaten on a regular basis in large quantities, i.e., at the FDA-recommended levels:

- Soy reduces our ability to assimilate essential nutrients like calcium, magnesium, copper, iron and zinc and it increases the body's requirement for vitamin D.
- Soy intake can cause growth problems and learning disabilities in children.
- Soy interferes with protein digestion and may cause pancreatic disorders.
- Soy phytoestrogens disrupt endocrine function and have the potential to cause infertility and to promote breast cancer in women.
- Soy phytoestrogens have been shown to cause hypothyroidism and may cause thyroid cancer.
- In infants, consumption of soy formula has been linked to autoimmune thyroid disease and the early onset of puberty.
- Industrial processing of soy protein results in the formation of cancer-causing agents.

- Industrial-processed soy foods contain high levels of aluminum, which is toxic to the nervous system and the kidneys.

Ladies, Soy Sucks and eating it can make you an infertile and overweight gas bomb with thyroid disease and breast cancer. Don't eat it and definitely don't feed it to babies or your man!

The next time you are offered plastic parading itself as "faux duck" or "nofurkey," I want you to stand up and shout: "No more fake food! Gimme the real thing!"

If you want more information on this topic, check out Kaayla Daniel's book *The Whole Soy Story*, or go to WestonAPrice.org and read more about the horrors of soy.

• DAIRY: IT DOES A BODY BAD! •

Dairy products in small doses—say, one slice of organic (preferably raw) cheese a day or a couple ounces of organic, full-fat (preferably nonhomogenized) milk in your organic coffee—aren't necessarily bad for us. However, many people have an intolerance to dairy—up to seventy-five percent of the world's population is lactose intolerant.

In Chinese Medicine, dairy products are right behind sugar on the phlegm spectrum. Think of a big glob of Philadelphia cream cheese or creamy Brie; as thick and viscous as it looks on your plate, that's how it remains once digested—making your digestive system grimy, gross and slow! Again, a little bit of dairy here and there isn't terrible. I mean, we all love indulging in the occasional Camembert or fresh whipped cream, and dairy on occasion is good for us. It's the overload of dairy products that is just no good for us. If you're eating, on a daily basis, something that your body cannot digest or break down— something that your body is potentially intolerant of—then over a period of time (say months or years) this indigestible matter takes up residence in your gut as layers and layers of phlegm. In CM theory, these layers of phlegm will line the entire digestive tract, inhibiting the absorption of nutrients. A body that isn't able to absorb nutrients from food thinks it's not being fed and it goes into "survival mode." And you don't want a body living in survival mode because it holds on to weight and shuts down certain functions it doesn't have the energy to carry out, like menstruation, metabolism or ovulation. The body can also become hostile to the phlegm accumulation, attacking it as it would foreign bacteria; this uncalled-for immune response results in what we in the Western world know as lactose intolerance.

Here's a quick little quiz for you.

Check off any of the following symptoms you experience more than once a week:

❏ Itchy, red rash or hives
❏ Eczema
❏ Nausea
❏ Diarrhea
❏ Bloating
❏ Sneezing
❏ Runny nose
❏ Wheezing
❏ Dull, heavy headache
❏ Fatigue

❏ Acne
❏ Black under-eye circles
❏ Vomiting
❏ Watery, itchy eyes
❏ Constipation
❏ Stomach cramping
❏ Gas
❏ Nasal congestion
❏ Under-eye puffiness

If you checked off even two of the above, I'm going to go out on a limb and say that you have big thick layers of phlegm traversing your gut. In fact, you, my dear, may be lactose intolerant. If you experience more than two of the symptoms, I recommend you cut out dairy entirely for a good solid month and give your body time to catch up. You can add it back in, slowly—over one month's time, one four-ounce serving per day—noting your symptoms and deciding if life without dairy may be better for you.

"Fine," you say, "maybe I'm lactose intolerant, but what about my bones? Don't I need to be drinking milk for the calcium? I don't want to be a hunched-over old lady!"

Lactose Intolerance vs. Dairy Allergy

When it comes to dairy, what most people refer to as a milk allergy is actually lactose intolerance. Lactose intolerance, which affects over fifty million Americans, is due to a deficiency of the enzyme lactase. Your body needs this enzyme to digest milk sugar, aka lactose. When you are lactase deficient, you cannot digest this sugar and it causes gas, bloating, stomach cramps, nausea, diarrhea and sometimes headaches.

When there's a true dairy allergy, your body is allergic to milk protein. This protein allergy is different from lactose intolerance in that it involves an immune system response. When you're allergic to milk protein, you will get symptoms similar to lactose intolerance, but you may also experience constipation, asthma, rashes, hives, sinus congestion, blood in your bowel movements and potentially anaphylactic shock!

To see if you have a true dairy allergy, ask your doctor to do some allergy testing on you.

Well, it's true, dairy products like milk offer us a good deal of calcium, which is important for strong and sexy bones. However, the Physicians Committee for Responsible Medicine points out: "There is much debate over whether long-term consumption of dairy products helps bones at all. A good deal of evidence suggests that it does not." Researchers at Harvard University found that adults who drank one glass of milk (or less) per week were at no greater risk of breaking a hip or forearm than were those who drank two or more glasses per week. Saving yourself from rickety old bones and hip replacements really just requires a good solid intake of foods naturally rich in calcium and vitamin D, as well as getting your ass to the gym.

Also, there's no scientific evidence that dairy intake prevents bone disease. The dairy industry's recommendation of three to four servings of dairy per day has not a hoof to stand on. There is not one study out there that has found that consuming more than one serving of dairy per day will prevent osteoporosis. However, there have been studies that have linked high dairy consumption to ovarian and prostate cancer.

"Wait, did you say I could get cancer from milk?"

Yes, I agree. It's a scary thought. Let me explain.

The cancer-causing agents in dairy are coming from the nonorganic, soy-fed (yes, our farm animals eat genetically modified and processed soy too!), nongrazing, miserable cows of America. These nonorganic-toxic-gross dairy products are chock-full of growth hormones and steroids, excess estrogens, soy, pesticides (which also contain estrogen) and antibiotics. That's the stuff that causes cancer.

GREAT CALCIUM FOOD SOURCES	SERVING SIZE	AMOUNT OF CALCIUM (MG)
Asparagus, boiled	1 cup	36
Basil, dried, ground	2 tsp.	60
Blackstrap molasses	2 tsp.	117
Broccoli, steamed	1 cup	75
Brussels sprouts, boiled	1 cup	56
Cabbage, shredded, boiled	1 cup	46
Celery, raw	1 cup	48
Cinnamon, ground	2 tsp.	56
Cloves, dried, ground	2 tsp.	28
Collard greens, boiled	1 cup	226
Cow's milk, full fat	1 cup	290
Fennel, raw, sliced	1 cup	43
Garlic	1 oz.	51
Goat's milk	1 cup	326
Green beans, boiled	1 cup	57
Kale, boiled	1 cup	93
Kelp	¼ cup	34
Mozzarella cheese	1 oz.	183
Mustard greens, boiled	1 cup	104
Mustard seeds	2 tsp.	39

Orange	1	52
Oregano, dried, ground	2 tsp.	47
Romaine lettuce	2 cups	40
Rosemary, dried	2 tsp.	28
Sesame seeds	¼ cup	351
Spinach, boiled	1 cup	245
Summer squash, cooked	1 cup	49
Swiss chard, boiled	1 cup	101
Turnip greens, cooked	1 cup	200
Thyme, dried, ground	2 tsp.	54
Yogurt	1 cup	447

Some scary facts on typical American dairy products:

- Dairy products from antibiotic- and steroid-pumped cows that are hormonally manipulated to produce three times more milk than the old-fashioned NOT hormonally manipulated cow contain toxins and cancer-causing agents.
- The pasteurization process, meant to protect us from harmful bacteria found in raw dairy products, also kills off beneficial bacteria that our body likes, destroys health-promoting nutrients and essential enzymes and makes dairy products indigestible. Furthermore, the lack of these enzymes puts stress on your pancreas to produce them itself. FYI: a woman with a stressed-out pancreas is more likely to get diabetes. To avoid the potential harms from pasteurization, you can try raw dairy products from certified healthy cows. In several states raw dairy is available commercially; in others, it can be bought directly from the farm. For more information on raw dairy and where to get it, go to realmilk.com.
- Any milk other than whole, full-fat milk is defatted, and it is not good for you, even if it's organic (although the organic defatted milks are better for you than the nonorganic ones). Listen up, ladies—fat is in milk for a reason: so that the body can absorb and use the vitamins and minerals milk

offers. After defatting milk, producers—even the organic guys—add synthetic vitamins back into the skim milk to "fortify" it. According to the *Physicians' Desk Reference*, only fifteen percent of synthetic nutrients are actually absorbable by our bodies. What's the point?

- The homogenization process of dairy was put in place to make your milk look pretty. You heard right: milk is homogenized for aesthetic purposes and that's it. But here's the juice: dairy's beauty is *definitely* only skin-deep. Homogenization, by mixing all the fat that's naturally occurring in dairy, changes the integrity of dairy products, preventing you from getting the benefit from the healthy fats found in dairy, and can actually be harmful to your health. Go for nonhomogenized dairy.

Dairy: it does a body bad. Have no more than one serving (about four ounces) of organic, hormone-free, antibiotic-free, nonhomogenized, steroid-free, full-fat and grass-fed dairy per day. Otherwise, you run the risk of getting cancer and diabetes.

A Word on Yogurt

Yogurt is fermented dairy, and like fermented soy, it's easier for our bodies to digest. Yogurt, because it's fermented, also contains health-promoting, immune-enhancing and life-extending bacterias (aka probiotics) that are oh so good for us. So, have a few servings of organic yogurt per week, and don't count it toward your dairy intake.

· SUGAR + BLEACH + ARSENIC = WHITE FLOUR ·

White flour is nothing more than wheat that's been adulterated with added sugar and bleach. It is disgusting and it will leave you obese, malnourished and prone to diabetes. Remember, added sugar contains arsenic; in that lovely slice of Wonder bread we have two majorly noxious substances: bleach and arsenic. Yummy!

"Oh, Aimee, I haven't eaten Wonder bread in ages."

I've got news for you. White flour isn't just in Wonder bread. It's in your morning bagel. It's in your lunch sandwich. It is in your weekly slice of pizza that you shouldn't be eating. It's in your fave upscale lunch spot's focaccia bread. It's in the pasta you eat twice weekly. It's even in your store-bought whole wheat bread. Yes, you heard me, white flour also goes by the names "enriched wheat flour" and "wheat flour."

Besides the noxious factor, white flour gives people obesity, heart disease and diabetes. Why? Bleach and processed sugar require insulin for the body to digest them. Insulin is a hormone secreted by the pancreas. Excess insulin makes for rapid weight gain and elevated triglycerides (fats that are often correlated with high cholesterol). What's even worse, because the body is getting little or no fuel from this bleached sugary arsenic stuff, it begins converting your already-existing muscle into energy. What this means is that if you are eating white flour regularly, toning your biceps at the gym is pointless because your poor body is so malnourished it's just going to eat up that muscle you are building and use it for the energy it needs to function. Ladies, if you want a hot, toned body, stop eating white flour!

A study published by the U.S. Department of Health found that if two groups of people are fed the exact same number of calories, but one group gets its calories from added sugars and processed products, while the other group consumes the calories in the form of whole grains, fruits, nuts and vegetables, the sugar group will gain weight, while the other will not. Duh!

Bottom line, white-flour products turn into sugar the second they enter your mouth. Reread the sugar section and then vow to never, ever eat white-flour products again. White flour should have gone out with the bad hairdos of the eighties.

White flour contains bleach and arsenic, makes you fat, gives you diabetes and heart disease and should be avoided like the plague.

All right, girls, now that I've told you about all the things you can't eat, let's move on to talking about what you actually can eat and feel good about.

6.

what the Hell can i actually Eat?

$\mathcal{R}$IGHT ABOUT NOW, you're probably thinking, "This lady is crazy. There is nothing I can eat!"

Darlin', there is plenty of food you can eat and actually feel good about.

"Really? Like what, water and twigs?"

No! Even better. I'll get into it in a moment; first let me tell you about Elizabeth.

Elizabeth came in to see me for what she suspected was a weak immune system, as she was always catching colds. She also had really, really low energy. Most mornings, even after eight solid hours of sleep she could barely get out of bed. Her hair was falling out, her nails were brittle and her skin was pale. She and her doctor both suspected a thyroid disorder, but her blood tests came back normal. As we talked, I found she was getting not only ample sleep but restful sleep; she wasn't very stressed-out by her job—in fact she liked her job—and she was generally a happy and easygoing person, although the nagging fatigue and constant colds were getting to her.

I also learned that for most of her life, she struggled with losing weight. However, over the last two years, through incorporating moderate exercise and following a strict "low-carb" and virtually fat-free diet, she lost twenty-five pounds. She was currently happy with her weight and I was too, as she didn't appear underweight and her weight loss was accomplished at a healthy pace.

However, I wasn't happy with her food choices.

For the last two years she'd been eating only "diet" foods like low-cal, low-carb frozen dinners, meal-replacement bars, diet soda, fat-free and sugar-free snacks and ice cream. She didn't eat any fruit because it had "too much sugar." She didn't cook any of her meals. The only vegetables she ate were the ones that came with her nightly frozen dinners.

Ladies, granted, Elizabeth lost weight, stuck to a plan and made it to her goal—which is awesome—but her diet was D-E-A-D and that's why she had zilch for energy and was constantly sick.

Is your diet dead too?

Do you eat nonfat, sugar-free, overly processed, nonnutritious foods? Are you constantly tired with dark circles under your eyes?

Girl, you need to stop eating dead food, because dead food, like I said in chapter 5, is made in some factory, loaded with preservatives and toxic chemicals and offers you absolutely squat for nutrition. These foods have no Qi, no life-engendering, antiaging, fertility-enhancing essence and absolutely no natural substances.

Remember the adage "You are what you eat"?

If you eat dead food, you're going to feel extremely tired and lifeless, look drawn and pale and have such a weak immune system that you get sick with each passing germ.

Ladies, you MUST eat nondead foods. I know you realize that your body is precious and that it wants to be alive and healthy—so treat it with respect and eat nutritionally packed, nondead foods!

"But I don't want to gain weight."

Eating nondead foods will not make you gain weight, because they will give you the proper nutrients and fats that your body needs to digest foods and maintain its metabolism. In fact, eating nondead food can actually help weight loss.

Eating "nondead" is not a two-week diet fad; it's a way of life. I didn't make it up. It's common sense—all you have to do is eat foods that are as close to their natural state as possible.

Huh?

When you look at a food or read a label, think, "How far did this travel from the tree it grew on, the ocean it swam in, the farm it was raised on or the soil it sprouted out of to get to my mouth?"

This means you're eating nothing that's been processed. No fast food. No "fat free." No "sugar free." No artificial sweeteners. No frozen entrées. Nothing that cooks instantly.

Elizabeth did it. She dropped all her processed, dead "diet" foods and began eating nondead foods. Now not only does she have enough energy to get through her day, but she actually makes it to the gym most mornings; she hasn't had a cold in months AND she hasn't gained any weight.

She did it by following my advice and becoming a label sleuth! You can do the same.

Because I've got news for you: your Vitaminwater, Balance Bar, non-fat soy mocha latte and favorite Tasti D-Lite frozen yogurt never ever saw soil or an ocean and they definitely didn't grow on a tree or a farm.

Darlin', I want you to eat a food only when you know exactly what it is you're eating; each item on the ingredient list should be recognizable and would be something that you could eat all on its own, like fresh fruit, organic stone-ground whole wheat, steamed veggies, organic butter and grilled hormone-free, antibiotic-free, humanely treated chicken. Get it?

For this chapter—so that I can offer you the savviest information—I have picked the brain of my favorite nutrition guru, Naomi Lewis. Naomi holds a master of science degree in nutrition from Bastyr University and a chef's training certification from Manhattan's Natural Gourmet Culinary Institute, and is certified in metabolic typing (check her out at eatberryhealthy.com). She is an amazingly well-informed woman who has, from my experience, a depth of nutritional knowledge incomparable with that of any other nutritionist I've worked with. Together with her overall nutritional advice and my specific CM dietary recommendations, this chapter will show you the ropes (and give you a one-week sample menu) on eating nutritionally sound and nondead.

First, I want to discuss some important "nondead" eating rules that you need to be clear on before you go food shopping and before you truly get on board with eating "nondead."

• ORGANIC IS IMPERATIVE •

Organic is NOT a conspiracy. It is one of the most important food movements of our lifetime. I know it's more expensive, but the way I look at it, pay now for organic food, or pay later for your poor health.

As a woman, you should be particularly keen on organic, as nonorganic foods are treated with pesticides, which are chemicals that contain (among other toxic things) xenoestrogens.

"Xeno what? Isn't she a warrior princess?"

These chemicals are far from the likes of a princess. Xenoestrogens mimic our own body's estrogen (like the plant estrogens in soy) and increase our chances of developing estrogen-dependent diseases in much the same way that soy foods do. Ladies, anything that adds more estrogen to our bodies is not a good thing.

What does organic mean?

Well, the USDA states in its Consumer Brochure: *Organic Food Standards and Labels: The Facts*:

"Organic food is produced by farmers who emphasize the use of renewable resources and the conservation of soil and water to enhance environmental quality for future generations. Organic meat, poultry, eggs, and dairy products come from animals that are given no antibiotics or growth hormones. Organic food is produced without using most conventional pesticides; fertilizers made with synthetic ingredients or sewage sludge; bioengineering; or ionizing radiation."

Let's break it down. Organic means:

- animals have not been treated with antibiotics (unless they get sick), growth hormones or feed made from animal by-products;
- animals have been fed organic feed for at least a year;
- the food hasn't been genetically modified, engineered or irradiated;
- the fertilizer that produced the "organic"-labeled products did not contain sewage sludge or synthetic ingredients;
- the produce hasn't been contaminated with synthetic chemicals used as pesticides;
- plants are grown in soil that has been organic for two or more years.

How do I know for sure that the food I'm buying really is organic?

True, some of the labeling on foods can be quite confusing. Let me explain to you what some of the labels actually mean:

- "One hundred percent organic": the product must contain one hundred percent organic ingredients.
- "Organic": at least ninety-five percent of ingredients are organically produced.
- "Made with organic ingredients": at least seventy percent of ingredients are organic. The remaining thirty percent must come from the USDA's approved list.
- "Free-range" or "free-roaming": this misleading term applies to chicken, eggs and other meat. The animal did not necessarily spend a good portion of its life outdoors. The rule states only that outdoor access be made available for "an undetermined period each day." U.S. government standards are weak in this area.

- "Natural" or "all-natural" does NOT mean organic. There is no standard definition for this term except with meat and poultry products. (USDA defines "natural" as not containing any artificial flavoring or colors, chemical preservatives or synthetic ingredients.) The claim is not verified. The producer or manufacturer alone decides whether to use it.

OK, so, to make it easier for you, I have compiled a list of the absolutely must-buy organic foods. These foods are in this list because if they are not organically grown, they are HIGHLY contaminated with pesticides. If you can't find these foods organically, skip 'em.

- Apples
- Cherries
- Grapes
- Raisins
- Nectarines
- Peaches
- Pears
- Apricots
- Raspberries
- Strawberries
- ALL fruit juice
- ALL dried fruits
- Lemons
- Limes
- Bell peppers
- Celery
- Potatoes
- Spinach
- Nuts
- Milk
- Eggs
- Meat
- Poultry

And here's a list of foods that have been shown to have a low pesticide load and are therefore A-OK to eat if they're not organic:

- Bananas
- Oranges
- Kiwis
- Mangoes
- Papaya
- Pineapples
- Asparagus
- Avocados
- Broccoli
- Cauliflower
- Corn (but be sure it's non-GM—I'll give you the lowdown on GMO below)

- Onions
- Peas (garden, snow and snap)

"But, Aimee, I *always* wash my fruits and veggies before I eat them! Do they still need to be organic?"

Gotcha. All of the info used to create the two lists you just read already considers that. Of course, washing and rinsing fresh produce will reduce levels of some pesticides, but it does not eliminate them. Peeling also reduces exposure, but valuable nutrients often go down the drain with the peel. The best way to reduce exposure to potentially harmful chemicals is to eat a varied diet, wash all produce and go organic.

Go to Environmental Working Group's Web site, ewg.org, for more information on the pesticide load of common fruits and veggies.

· BEWARE OF CLONES! ·

Genetically modified (GM) foods and organisms are everywhere!

Girl, if you were to randomly pick an item off your grocery store's shelves, you have a seventy percent chance of picking a food with GM ingredients. This is because at least seven out of every ten items in your local grocery have been genetically modified. Jeez Louise!

The genetic modification, or genetic engineering, of foods started out with the best of intentions: to protect our crops and maintain an adequate food supply for the ever-growing world population. Sounds great! Well, not really. You see, what started out as a decent idea (not really, though) has turned our food supply into the land of the walking DEAD clones. Food containing GM substances is synthetic and unnatural. Don't eat it. GM substances, besides being very, very far from natural, are increasing the incidences of food allergies and antibiotic-resistant bacteria in our population. What's even scarier is that the potential long-term human-health hazards they impose are still unknown.

I urge you to follow these four simple steps and decrease your consumption of GM foods:

- Reduce or eliminate processed foods in your diet.
- Read produce and food labels. Soybeans and corn make up the largest portion of GM crops. Ingredients made from these foods include high-fructose corn syrup (and all the other "sugar in disguise" names I gave in chapter 5), corn flour and cornmeal, dextrin, starch, margarine, anything that contains soy—including soy oil, soy protein isolate and tofu products. Don't eat any of these products!
- Buy organic food. By definition, food that is certified organic must be free from all GM organisms, produced without artificial pesticides and fertilizers and derived from an animal raised without antibiotics, growth hormones or other noxious drugs. Just an FYI: grass-fed beef comes from cows that are never fed GM corn feed.
- Look at produce stickers. The PLU code on stickers for conventionally grown fruit consists of four numbers, organically grown fruit has five numbers beginning with the number nine, and GM fruit has five numbers beginning with the number eight.

For more information on this topic, read *Genetic Roulette* by Jeffrey M. Smith.

· SOMETHING SMELLS FISHY ·

When it comes to seafood, it's difficult to make simple dietary recommendations; from whether wild fish is better or just as good as farm-raised fish to how much tuna one can eat—the consumer information is constantly changing. One of the major issues here is that no USDA organic certification exists for seafood—so producers can make any claim they want. Basically fishmongers can call any seafood "organic" even if it's loaded with poisonous mercury, heavy metals, chemicals and PCBs and harmful bacteria. Another major issue is the ever-increasing environmental pollutants that are affecting our waters and our seafood.

So what's a girl to do?

For me, I find that Monterey Bay Aquarium (mbayaq.org) and Environmental Working Group (ewg.org) have the best, up-to-date, what-fish-to-eat-or-not-to-eat information out there. And I'm going to pass their advice on to you: eat a wide variety of sustainable fish— eat them mostly wild, although there are some farm-raised fish that are safe too—that have a moderate or low level of poisonous toxins. Here's the most current list I have of such safe-to-eat fish:

- Rainbow trout (U.S. farm-raised is considered safe)
- Sardines
- Oysters
- Mussels
- Anchovies
- Crawfish
- Herring
- Bay scallops
- Wild Alaska salmon
- Clams

Now, keep in mind, the above list is a general guideline for the entire nation. The safety of fish does vary from location to location. For an up-to-date, safe-to-eat-or-not-to-eat list of seafood where you live (or may be traveling to), go to Monterey Bay Aquarium's seafoodwatch page at www.mbayaq.org/cr/cr_seafoodwatch/download.asp. Check it out. You'll be relieved to find that there are plenty of great local fish choices you can make beyond the limited national list of safe-to-eat fish. I use this link all the time before I hit the grocery store or head out for a seafood dinner!

. . .

A WORD ABOUT TUNA

When it comes to albacore (white) tuna, because of the high levels of poisonous-to-our-body mercury it contains, the rule of thumb is to eat one serving (one serving = the size of your palm = four or so ounces) no more than twice a month. As far as tuna steaks (bluefin, yellowfin and bigeye) are concerned, they definitely contain a good amount of mercury—you shouldn't eat tuna steaks any more than once a month. And if you're pregnant, or trying to get pregnant, steer clear of tuna, and ANY fish that has a moderate-to-high level of mercury, as the mercury these fish contain is a very dangerous neurotoxin that can cross the umbilical cord and harm your baby.

In addition, the Environmental Working Group recommends that children younger than twelve shouldn't eat more than six ounces of albacore tuna a week.

Regarding canned tuna, chunk light tuna (which consists primarily of skipjack fish) is your best option because it's lower in mercury than white, or albacore, tuna.

A great online site to purchase safe-to-eat fish, particularly canned light tuna and salmon, is Vital Choice (vitalchoice.com). They also sell organic nuts, seeds, oils and teas.

Eggs do not give you high cholesterol.

"What?!"

Yes, eggs are high in cholesterol. They are also high in several other important nutrients—notably, lecithin—that help your body balance the cholesterol content and keep cholesterol circulating in your blood rather than allowing it to form deposits in your arteries. These other nutrients found in eggs also help your liver produce bile, which is critical for digestion, absorbing fat and eliminating crap. And in case you didn't know, cholesterol is an imperative substance in your body; it helps produce hormones, vitamin D and bile so that you can digest fat. A lot of times, a body that is deprived of healthy fats that contain cholesterol will actually INCREASE its cholesterol production. That's how badly your body needs cholesterol.

Researchers at Harvard who followed 115,000 people for eight or more years found that eating one egg per day did not have a harmful effect on their cholesterol levels, nor did it increase their risk of heart disease or stroke.

Additionally, *Mother Earth News* conducted their own research project; they compared conventional, confined, help-I-can't-move chicken eggs with free-roaming, ahhh-isn't-that-a-nice-breeze chicken eggs and found that eggs from free-range chickens contain one-third less cholesterol and one-fourth less saturated fat!

Listen to this: according to a study from Pennington Biomedical Research Center in Baton Rouge, Louisiana, overweight women who ate eggs for breakfast lost twice as much weight as women who started their days with bagels. Researchers say the protein in eggs increases satiety and decreases hunger, helping women eat fewer calories throughout the day.

Have six to eight free-range chicken eggs with their yolks per week.

• • •

· EAT FAT! ·

Ladies, nonfat girls get more wrinkles and have saggy boobs! I'm not saying to go out and eat loads of trans fats; I'm saying eat a wide variety of good healthy fats. Fat should be your friend (especially if you are that lucky girl who has a hard time gaining weight and tends to be lean). Fat is good for nutrient absorption, concentration, energy level, hormonal regulation and fertility, shiny hair and strong nails. Eat it in the form of nuts, avocados, flaxseeds, olive oil, eggs, meat, coconut oil, ghee, organic butter and fatty fish like salmon.

Packaged fat-free cookies, ice cream and the like are often processed, dead, chemically treated and lacking important nutrients that your body needs to look great and feel good. Do yourself and your health a huge favor and DON'T eat them. The best fat-free foods are the ones that are naturally fat-free . . . you know, like fresh fruit and veggies.

For more information on this topic, check out the book *Know Your Fats* by Mary Enig.

· EAT MEAT! ·

Yup, you heard me. Eat meat! Chicken, lamb, duck, beef, pork, turkey, buffalo, elk, venison—you name it, eat it. Chinese Medicine touts meat and uses it medicinally because it's one of the best essence-generating foods going; it builds Qi, nourishes blood and helps keep your body strong and healthy. Animal meats are loaded with all the nutrients and protein any high-functioning body could want. Obviously, I'm not recommending you eat a big fatty rib-eye steak every night for dinner, but I am saying to have three or four ounces of hormone-free, antibiotic-free, organically raised lean meat five to six days a week. And remember, grass-fed beef is the best. Eat it—your body will thank you.

· EAT FOODS THAT ARE IN SEASON ·
AND LOCALLY GROWN

Girl, get to the nearest farmers' market as often as possible! Support your local farmers—it's great for your community.

"Why should I buy locally grown food?"

Because it's fresher than any comparable food you'll find in your supermarket, not to mention that it's tastier and healthier. And buying food at your local farmers' market is good for your local economy—and it puts money directly in the pockets of the families that farmed the food.

A great Web site to find farmers' markets, family farms and other sources of food grown in your area is LocalHarvest.org.

"Is local better than organic?"

Well, here's the thing: much of the time locally grown food is organic, but the farms are too small and the process too expensive for the local farmer to get the certified-organic label. The best thing to do is to talk to the farmers themselves and find out how they run their farm.

Eating locally also means that you are eating foods that are in season for your part of the country. That's a good thing. Mother Nature knew what she was doing when she set this place up. In CM theory, eating foods that are in season means you are in sync with your environment. When it's winter, it's not a good idea to be eating watermelon, just like in the summer very few people crave a beef and veggie stew. Get it?

And then there's the whole environmental burden from foods—organic or not—that are shipped all over our country in big ol' gas-guzzling trucks. When you buy locally, that burden isn't an issue.

In my opinion, shopping locally is a great option and it just feels good to know that you're supporting some small family farm, but the bottom line is that you don't want to eat anything that's loaded with pesticides. Just be sure to eat foods that are organic and in season.

• VODKA ROCKS! •

Quite the name for a section in a get-healthy book, huh? Listen, I'd be a hypocrite if I told you not to drink. And hypocrites aren't cool. Instead I'm going to tell you what to drink.

Drink vodka. In moderation, of course.

My cocktail of choice is vodka and seltzer water (or sodium-free soda water). You heard me right. Vodka is typically distilled dozens, if not hundreds, of times per batch. Fortunately for us, the nineteenth-century invention of multiple distillations in a single cylinder made it economical to achieve unprecedented levels of purity. Sure, vodka is forty percent alcohol, but the other sixty percent is water. This libation is one of the cleanest out there because when a grain, fruit or vegetable is distilled, it contains NO added sugar. Mix it with seltzer water, and it remains clean (because, again, there is NO added sugar). Add a couple of lime or lemon wedges (I've even had watermelon slices, yummy!). Voilà, you have quite a refreshing and sugarless cocktail. I tend to think potato vodkas (like Chopin) are the best, mainly because the other two common bases are wheat and soy, which are both common allergens.

Now, I'm not saying to go out and have a dozen vodka cocktails. But don't deprive yourself of a vice you may love. Just choose wisely. And at all costs, avoid mixing your vodka with an added-sugar juice or soda!!

• THE BEST WAY TO PREPARE YOUR FOOD •

When it comes to food preparation, it's important to know what to do. Here's a little cheat sheet for you:

- **EGGS:** hard-boil, soft-boil or panfry. Use organic butter, ghee or coconut oil to cook. DO NOT use olive oil to cook eggs (I'll tell you why in a sec).

- **CHICKEN:** grill, bake or cook on the stove top. Use organic butter, ghee, coconut oil or olive oil (when baking or using a low flame on the stove top) to cook.
- **FISH:** broil, steam or grill. Use organic butter, ghee, or olive or coconut oil to cook.
- **MEAT:** pan-sear, grill or broil. Use organic butter, ghee or coconut oil to cook. DO NOT use olive oil to cook meat.
- **BEANS:** you should always soak your beans before you cook them. Soaking them breaks down the naturally occurring sugars in beans. It's these sugars that make beans hard to digest and give you gas. So soak your beans for six to eight hours (or overnight) before cooking. In a large saucepan, soak the beans in three times as much water as beans, and add one tablespoon of lemon juice or one teaspoon of apple-cider vinegar. If there's no time for a six-hour soak, no worries—you can quick-soak. Cover beans with water, bring to a boil, then turn off the heat and let sit for an hour or two. To make beans most digestible, always drain the soaking liquid and cook in fresh water.
- **NUTS AND GRAINS:** listen, I know this is overkill, but there is a proper way to prepare your nuts and grains. Whether you do it—hey, that's up to you. But nuts and grains contain numerous enzyme inhibitors that hamper their ability to be properly digested and block your body's absorption of essential nutrients. So if you want to get the most out of your nuts and grains, you gotta soak 'em. Soak your nuts in filtered water with two teaspoons of sea salt for six to eight hours, then dry them in your oven at 150 degrees for twelve to twenty-four hours. Soak (or sprout) your grains. First rinse them with water, then soak them in a mixture of water, one teaspoon of sea salt and a splash of lemon juice or raw apple-cider vinegar for seven hours (or overnight, but don't refrigerate them). Naomi says it's easiest to soak your grains in the pot that you will cook them in, using a two-to-one ratio of water to grain.

> ### *Beware: Cooking with Olive Oil*
>
> Olive oil is great for dressing salads, for baking and for cooking fish, but when it comes to cooking other foods that require a high temperature, olive oil isn't the best choice. At high temperatures olive oil (like flaxseed oil) goes rancid, offers us no nutritional value and can be harmful to our health!
>
> Here's a good rule of thumb: if you're cooking with more than a medium flame on the stove top, DON'T use olive oil.
>
> Use coconut or sesame oil, butter or ghee instead.

• ONE WEEK'S "NONDEAD" SAMPLE MENU •

All right, ladies, here's the juice. Keep in mind this seven-day menu is just a template—an example—of the types of things you can and should be eating. I know it's a bit overwhelming to think about eating entirely clean, organic, sugar free, full fat, non-DEAD and soyless, but you can do it. Following the "nondead" way of life isn't hard, but it is going to require you to prepare some of your foods and to be completely aware of the origin of each and every morsel you put in that precious mouth of yours. Of course, I'm stickin' with the "everything in moderation" motto here too. So, girl, "Be Mod." Meaning, eighty to eighty-five percent of the time eat clean, organic and nondead, and the other fifteen to twenty percent of the time you can stray a little. So once in a while if you eat out and have nonorganic chicken, I'm not going to hunt you down and beat you up. I promise! I just want you to be conscious of what you are eating, and when faced with a limited menu, make the best choice possible for your health.

"But, Aimee, what am I going to do for lunch during the workweek?"

Brown-bag it, babe!

"I don't have time to make my lunch every morning!"

If I can do it, you can do it. Really, it's not hard. Prepare food on Sunday for a week's worth of lunch. You can make soups or stews; prebake sweet potatoes; grill some steak, chicken breasts, shrimp or salmon for a salad; have homemade guac in the fridge; cut up some veggies and roast them; use your food processor that's been collecting dust for the last two years and make some fresh hummus; hard-boil a dozen eggs and keep them in your fridge for a quick energy-boosting snack. Get it? Cooking is also übertherapeutic and fun! Get out your grandma's cookbooks and get back your health.

What If I Have to Dine Out Frequently for Work?

Eating clean and nondead while dining out can be tough. Here's a good rule of thumb: be sure your breakfast and lunch are clean and nondead. This way, by following the Be Mod rule (eating clean and nondead eighty to eighty-five percent of the time, straying fifteen to twenty percent of the time), you can have four dinners a week that aren't completely clean and nondead. I mean, don't overindulge in the likes of fried chicken, heaps of mashed potatoes and chocolate mousse. Still, try and make the best choice possible, even if that choice is not one hundred percent clean and nondead.

Sweety, this whole nondead eating thing is totally doable. You can do it!

Go out and stock up on organic snacks like yogurt, nut butter, fruit and nuts. Make yourself a big batch of trail mix and separate it into little Baggies, then throw one in your gym bag each day for an after-work snack. Or take a yogurt to work with you for a midmorning snack. Throw a peach in your purse for later. Bring some carrots and peanut or almond butter with you to work. Poor food choices arise when we are starved and aren't prepared—so be prepared. Honestly, it'll require a couple hours of your time on a Sunday to live a healthier life all week. Your health is worth an hour or two on a Sunday afternoon, isn't it?

And for when you're feeling lazy—scope out the healthy, organic lunch spots that you can feel good about eating at. They're out there. Ask around. Also, online Greenopia.com is a great place to look.

Keep in Mind

A serving size is
- for meat, fish or poultry, the size of your palm
- for rice or pasta, the size of a tennis ball.

Here goes the seven-day menu. . . . Remember, all foods here are to be organic, fresh and "nondead"!

DAY 1

- **BREAKFAST:** two scrambled eggs with tomato and fresh basil, a piece of bacon and a slice of whole-grain bread

- **LUNCH:** mixed mesclun-green salad with wild salmon, onions, green beans, olives, olive oil and vinegar

- **SNACK:** a banana and two handfuls of almonds or cashews

- **DINNER:** baked chicken with fresh herbs, sautéed kale with garlic and a sweet potato with a touch of butter

DAY 2

- **BREAKFAST:** one hard-boiled egg and a cup of steel-cut oats with blueberries, walnuts and a teaspoon of raw honey

- **LUNCH:** whole-grain tortilla roll-up with hummus, sprouts, grated carrots and arugula

- **SNACK:** Lärabar or a handful of nuts and a piece of fruit

- **DINNER:** beef tenderloin with sautéed bok choy, garlic and spinach and side of brown rice. Flavor with juice from half a lemon and a dash of sea salt.

sejal's Homemade Hummus

My friend Sejal makes the best freakin' hummus ... and it's so easy to make. Here's her recipe:

3 cups drained cooked organic chickpeas (you can use canned organic chickpeas)

2 medium cloves garlic

¼ teaspoon crushed red pepper (optional)

½ cup tahini

2 tablespoons water

4 tablespoons organic lemon juice, to taste

4 tablespoons organic extra-virgin olive oil

1 tablespoon chopped parsley leaves

¼ teaspoon paprika

In your food processor, puree the chickpeas, garlic cloves, red pepper, tahini, water, half the lemon juice and half the olive oil until smooth, stopping to scrape down the sides as needed. Taste and adjust the seasoning by adding salt and additional lemon juice, if necessary, to your liking. Transfer to a wide shallow bowl for serving and use the back of a serving spoon to form a well in the center of the hummus. Drizzle with the remaining olive oil and sprinkle the top with the parsley and paprika. Voilà!

• • •

DAY 3

- **BREAKFAST:** one cup of cow, goat or sheep yogurt sprinkled with ground flaxseeds and a coconut-milk smoothie with banana, blueberries and strawberries

- **LUNCH:** watercress salad with grilled chicken, avocado, mushrooms (shiitake, maitake or black), goat's milk feta cheese, olive oil and vinegar. Flavor with some fresh ground pepper.

- **SNACK:** a slice of whole-grain or rice bread with almond butter and a cup of honeydew melon (or any other fruit that's in season)

- **DINNER:** sautéed fillet of sole with shallots and leeks, roasted red potatoes with rosemary and olive oil and steamed asparagus. Garnish with the juice from half a lemon.

Naomi's Root-veggie Medley

4 beets
2 sweet potatoes
3 turnips
1 parsnip
2 cloves chopped garlic
¼ cup organic olive oil
Sea salt and pepper to taste

Cut veggies into small pieces, add in the garlic, mix with olive oil, sprinkle with sea salt and pepper. Bake at 400 degrees till veggies are crispy, around 45 minutes.

Voilà! You have veggies for the week!

• • •

DAY 4

- **BREAKFAST:** two eggs over easy with one lamb, turkey or chicken sausage

- **LUNCH:** a bowl of Health Valley organic soup (or Wolfgang Puck makes great organic soup too!) with one piece whole-grain or rice bread or some whole-grain or rice crackers

- **SNACK:** cow, goat or sheep yogurt with goji berries and walnuts

- **DINNER:** grilled wild salmon with sautéed maitake mushrooms and garlic and a serving of root-veggie medley

DAY 5

- **BREAKFAST:** one fried egg with a slice of stone-ground whole wheat toast and a grapefruit

- **LUNCH:** mixed green salad with kidney beans, corn, avocado, tomato, olives, olive oil and vinegar

- **SNACK:** a Garden of Life or Dr. Weil's bar, or some Newman's Own organic pretzels and guac

- **DINNER:** hamburger on whole-grain bun with lettuce, tomato and onion, baked French fries and sautéed spinach

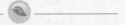

Here's how I manage to eat nondead eighty to eighty-five percent of my life.

I pretty much *ALWAYS* cook my own breakfast. So I make sure to always have organic, free-range eggs in my apartment, along with organic full-fat yogurt, fresh organic fruit and organic steel-cut oatmeal. This way I have a good breakfast selection.

If I'm running late one morning, I'll just grab a yogurt (either Stonyfield or Oikos) or two hard-boiled eggs and some fruit and go. Or I just throw some all-natural and organic peanut butter on a slice of organic whole-grain or spelt bread and eat it while I'm running out the door—not ideal, but sometimes you gotta do it. But for the most part, I try to put aside the extra ten to fifteen minutes to prepare, sit down and enjoy a healthy, organic breakfast. Yes, it takes only an extra ten to fifteen minutes to prepare and eat breakfast!

If I know I'm going to be in the office all day, I pack my lunch. Usually, on Sundays I bake three or four organic, free-range chicken breasts (then slice them so they're ready to throw on a salad or over some quinoa); I grill one or two grass-fed beef patties (or I make meatballs); I also make some egg salad, guacamole, hard-boiled eggs and hummus. I always make sure I have some organic fresh salad leaves in the fridge. So depending on what I'm in the mood for, I either make a quick salad with grilled chicken, throw some meatballs in a Tupperware to go or throw some hummus into a whole-grain wrap with some salad leaves, onion and carrots. I'll bring some guac and rice crackers or organic whole-grain pretzels and some fruit for a snack. And I always have a container of my homemade organic trail mix at the office in case I need something to pick at. If I'm in a rush and didn't have time to grab a snack, I'll swing by a deli and pick up some almonds and a banana or an orange or some cut-up pineapple or mango, as I know those are great nonorganic choices. Or I grab an always-organic Lärabar.

For dinner, I try to cook at home with fresh fish, healthy organic meats, organic veggies and grains, but I do enjoy dining out and I don't deprive myself of that. Sometimes it's tough to eat completely clean and nondead when I'm dining out. So I always apply my "Be Mod" rule (eating clean and nondead eighty to eighty-five percent of the time). If I have time to plan, I check out which fish is safe to eat on mbayaq.org and try to order one of those. A lot of times I eat out at restaurants where I know that they serve fresh organic produce and meats—if I'm unsure, I ask a lot of questions. Some of my major rules: I always get sauces on the side, I never order anything in a cream sauce and I ask for a veggie that is safe if it's not organic (like broccoli, cauliflower and asparagus).

And then there are times when I go all out and "Be Mod" and I order a burger and fries. Hey—you gotta live a little!

Aimee's famous guac

2 avocados, cut into ¼ inch cubes
1 tomato
¼ red onion
2 cloves garlic, finely chopped
2 dashes balsamic vinegar
Juice from ½ lemon

In a large bowl, using a fork, mash all the ingredients together. That's it!

DAY 6

- **BREAKFAST:** yogurt with granola and mixed berries

- **LUNCH:** sliced steak with steamed broccoli and peppers over a red cabbage salad. Garnish with cracked pepper.

- **SNACK:** two nectarines and two handfuls of homemade trail mix

- **DINNER:** chicken stir-fry with bok choy, onion, garlic, mushrooms (maitake, shiitake and black), cashews and brown rice

DAY 7

- **BREAKFAST:** two scrambled eggs with goat cheese and spinach and one piece spelt bread

- **LUNCH:** whole-grain tortilla roll-up with canned light tuna salad, capers, onion, celery and mixed greens

- **SNACK:** hummus and carrots

- **DINNER:** baked chicken with fresh parsley and thyme, corn on the cob and sautéed green beans with sliced almonds

When you're starved and in a pinch, here are some foods that you can find in your local corner deli that you can actually feel good about eating!

Healthy health bars: Lärabar, Garden of Life, Dr. Weil by Nature's Path, Wings of Nature and BumbleBar. Yes, these bars have a lot of sugar, but remember, it's naturally occurring sugars and your body metabolizes them differently than added sugars. These "fast-food" bars are as close to nature as you can get.

When you can't find organic nuts or seeds, choose almonds, walnuts, sunflower seeds and pumpkin seeds.

When you can't find organic fruit, choose bananas, grapefruit, honeydew melon, watermelon, papayas, kiwis, mangoes, pineapples, blueberries and tangerines.

Organic snack foods include: Newman's Own organic pretzels, Suzie's crackers, Mary's Gone Crackers crackers and Shiloh Farms organic popcorn.

Snacks You Can Bring from Home to the Office

- Hard-boiled eggs
- Peanut or almond butter (all-natural, organic, nothing added) and celery
- Organic hummus and carrots
- Homemade trail mix: buy some organic raisins, sunflower seeds, goji berries, pumpkin seeds, peanuts and almonds, and mix them all together; take a small Baggie of the mixture with you to work.
- Homemade guacamole and whole-grain or rice crackers

• • •

· "HEALTH" FOODS YOU DEFINITELY ·
SHOULDN'T BE EATING

I know this chapter is about what you CAN eat, but I just need to point out some of the so-called health foods that you should NOT eat.

- Any overly processed "meal replacement" or "health" bar that's loaded with added sugars, contains synthetic and unabsorbable vitamins and genetically modified soy products, and is not one hundred percent organic. Here's a list of the most common ones out there—but I'm sure there are some I am missing. So it's ultimately up to you: read ingredients, be a label sleuth!

  - Luna
  - Kashi bars
  - Odwalla
  - Balance
  - The Zone
  - Protria

  - Advantage
  - Myoplex
  - Genisoy
  - Ultrasoy
  - EAS
  - Nature's Plus Energy Bar

- Vitaminwater or any "sugar water" like Gatorade—unless, of course, you're a professional athlete or training for an athletic event (like a marathon or a triathlon) and need to replenish your body with electrolytes ... AFTER a long workout. That's why most of these drinks are called "sports drinks": they are not meant for daily beverage consumption; they are meant for athletes after exercise and even then in moderation.
- Processed lunch meats (get nitrate-free ones instead!).

· THE LOWDOWN ON ·
NUTRITIONAL SUPPLEMENTS

This section is here because a lot of us take supplements to help our bodies function better. Personally, I'm not a huge fan of oversupplementation, but I am a fan of supplementing with certain nutrients we can't get from our diets. First and foremost, I believe that we should be able to get most of our nutrients from the foods we eat (especially when eating a diet like I just mapped out for you). However, with the current state of our precious American soil—organic or not—our foods aren't nearly as nutritious as they once were. Last year I heard a lecture by Patrick Shelley, the founder and CEO of NutriHarmony, and what he said shook me to the core. In a nutshell, he said that in 1960 a plateful of food (meat, potatoes and veggies) gave one all the nutrients he or she needed for that day. In today's world, with the state of our soil and the amount of pesticides and chemicals used on our foods, you would need to eat an entire wheelbarrow full of that same food to get all the nutrients you'd need for the day.

A wheelbarrow? OMG!

Bottom line: with the state of our foods and our ghastly typical American diets, we need to supplement certain nutrients. This need for supplementation brings us to a whole new issue. How nutritiously sound are the vitamins we buy, and where do they come from? The 2006 *Physicians' Desk Reference* states that only eight to fifteen percent of any synthesized nutritional supplement (i.e., those made in a laboratory) is actually absorbable by the human body! What this means is that vitamins that are not made from whole-food sources are a complete waste of your money. Unfortunately most of the vitamins on the market are made in laboratories where individual nutrients are created and then packed into nice little capsules for you to swallow. The problem here is that things like vitamin A or B_6 do not exist in nature all by themselves. Vitamins coexist with other vitamins and phytonutrients. In order for the human body to assimilate these vitamins and use them to optimize bodily functions, they need to present themselves to us with their other vitamin and phytonutrient friends. So synthetic vitamins, although made with the best intentions, actually offer us no nutritional value and are a complete waste of our money.

And then there are whole-food vitamins. Not "Whole Foods" as in the store; "whole food" as in whole food—the way it occur nature.

These vitamins deliver nutrients with their vitamin and phytonutrient friends so that we can absorb them and use them for all they're worth. There are some really good companies out there making some killer vitamins that are nearly one hundred percent absorbable. Some of my favorite brands are NutriHarmony, Garden of Life, Dr. Ron's, Radiant Life and New Chapter (they use non-GMO soy in some of their vitamin formulations). But again, I don't overrecommend supplements. I think we should do our best to get our nutrients from our foods. I do, however, urge most everyone to take the following three supplements to assist them in achieving optimal health.

1. **COD-LIVER OIL:** I recommend supplementing with cod-liver oil because it is the richest source of omega-3 essential fatty acids (EFAs). These EFAs play an important role in helping our bodies produce and regulate hormones, manage inflammation and maintain a high-functioning brain and nervous system. Sounds awesome! Not only awesome, but imperative—but here's the thing: our bodies cannot produce these omega-3 EFAs on their own. In order to get these nutrients in, we often need to take an omega-3-rich supplement. Because when women don't have enough omega-3 EFAs in their diet, they usually have bad PMS, menstrual cramps, irregular periods, hormonally related acne and weight gain, infertility and pregnancy-related problems. Ahh!

   I know what you're wondering. Why can't I just get these omega-3 EFAs from my diet?

   Well, you could. Omega-3 EFAs are commonly found in cold-water fish, flaxseeds, walnuts, canola oil, whole grains, legumes, nuts and green leafy vegetables. But here's the glitch: the typical American diet contains a heckuva lot more omega-6 EFAs (found in foods like grains, plant-based oils, eggs and poultry) than omega-3, and a body in optimal health should have equal amounts. So the key is to supplement with omega-3.

   In addition, cod-liver oil is a great source of vitamins A

and D. Vitamin A helps your eyes adjust to light changes and keeps your eyes and skin hydrated, and vitamin D is essential for maintaining good healthy bones. Another great source of Vitamin D is direct sunlight. So in the warmer months, if you are getting a lot of sun, then I recommend you take fish oil rather than cod-liver oil, but other than that, take cod-liver oil.

Purchase this in capsule form because the oil tastes not so great and you probably won't take it. The goal is to get in two to three thousand milligrams per day of the oil; take with food. If you experience loose bowel movements after taking it, cut the dosage back by a thousand milligrams. The best-quality, mercury-free, happy-fish brands I recommend:

- **In stores**—Garden of Life CODmega and Nordic Naturals Arctic D cod-liver oil or Ultimate Omega with D3
- **Online**—Dr. Ron's Pure High Vitamin Blue Ice cod-liver oil (drrons.com), Radiant Life Premier Quantum Norwegian Cod Liver Oil (4radiantlife.com) and Green Pasture's Blue Ice, High Vitamin cod-liver oil (green-pasture.org)

2. **SPIRULINA: spirulina** is a freshwater blue-green alga that's nearly three and a half BILLION years old; it's a tremendously rich source of protein, EFAs and vitamins like B_1, B_2, B_3, B_6, B_9, C, D and E. Bottom line: I love this stuff because it is full of age-fighting antioxidants, boosts your immune system and, in a nutshell, is amazing for your overall health!

Spirulina comes in tablet, capsule or powder form. Personally, I take it in capsule form because I find that the easiest. Whichever brand you decide to get, take it as directed on the bottle. My all-time favorite, top-notch brands of spirulina:

- **In stores**—Nutrex Hawaiian Organic Spirulina or Garden of Life Perfect Food
- **Online**—NutriHarmony Garden and the Greens

3. **PROBIOTICS:** the word "probiotic" means "for life." Probiotics are the good bacteria found in your digestive tract. Taking a probiotic supplement helps to maintain the natural balance of good and bad bacteria in your body, improves your digestion, boosts your immune system and just makes you healthier.

I'm sure you've heard of probiotics before—they're often touted as natural components of certain foods like Dannon's Activia yogurt. Like all nutritional supplements, probiotics come in many shapes and sizes and some forms are just plain ol' not worth an inkling of your time or money. The key thing about ingesting a probiotic is that it needs to survive the harsh acidity in your stomach and make it to your small intestine so that it can actually give you some of its benefits. So eating foods enriched with a probiotic is pointless, because they will get digested in the stomach and you won't get any benefit (not to mention that you'd have to eat ten yogurts to get the amount of probiotic found in one capsule).

With that said, I have only one brand of probiotic that I recommend: Culturelle. There is a ton of science backing up the efficacy of this brand and the good, healthy bacteria it delivers.

Of course, there are other great brands out there (like Genestra's HMF Forte), but the science behind Culturelle makes me feel great about recommending it.

Take as directed. You can find it in most health-food stores.

Ladies, next, we're going to move on to, I'm sure, some very important topics to you ... managing your PMS, controlling what feels like hormonal mayhem in your body and enhancing your fertility factors. Woo hoo!

preparing
the palace

$\mathcal{S}$ARAH, A PEDIATRIC nurse, called me for an emergency appointment—she had a "killer" migraine and the Imitrex prescribed to her wasn't working. At our first visit, Sarah was in so much pain, we really didn't chat much. I helped alleviate her migraine and a week later she came back for a follow-up appointment. It was then that I learned more about her migraine history: she suffered with premenstrual migraines from the onset of her period at age fourteen. At age sixteen she went on the birth control pill, not because she was sexually active, but to control her migraines. On the Pill, she still suffered with intense PMS, "viselike" menstrual cramps and heavy periods, and yes, she still got the premenstrual migraines, but they were less frequent and less debilitating—one Imitrex usually took care of them.

At our second meeting, she told me that after sixteen years she had recently stopped taking the Pill; it had been six weeks since her last period, and she had suffered two "killer" migraines and was feeling very irritable, bloated and emotional. She was concerned that when her period finally came, her premenstrual symptoms and migraines would make her life miserable, but moreover she was anxious to get her period, as she wanted to start trying to have a baby and feared she might be infertile. She asked if I thought I could help her get pregnant.

I said, "First we need to prepare your palace."

She looked at me like I had two heads and I'm sure she was thinking the same thing you are: "Palace?! Aimee, I thought we were talking about health, not interior design!"

Aha! Don't you see by now that your interior design and your health are one and the same? Ladies, the palace I'm referring to is not the Helmsley Palace Hotel. I'm talking about your baby-making machinery—your female reproductive system, including your uterus, ovaries, fallopian tubes and cervix.

In Chinese Medicine we refer to the female reproductive system as a "palace" because it is the richest place on earth. Your "palace" is the foundation of all that is: it houses and nurtures the building blocks for life. Girl, your reproductive system is Eden and it should be a majestic and welcoming baby-growing paradise; it should be ovulating and menstruating regularly, with minimal PMS and cramping. Sarah's history of intense PMS and "viselike" menstrual cramps coupled with her "killer" migraines and the fact that she hadn't yet menstruated since being off the Pill all point to the fact that her female reproductive system—her "palace"—is definitely not functioning optimally. Her hormones are completely out of balance and it could be months before she has a normal ovulation. The chances of her "palace" being a majestic and welcoming baby-growing paradise, right now, are pretty slim. That's why I need to first help Sarah prepare her palace. Get it?

You see, when I use the term *preparing the palace*, I mean, let's get the interior design of your female reproductive system into a proficient baby-making nirvana. Let's get your PMS and other hormone-related issues like premenstrual migraines, raging emotions, acne, breast tenderness, bloating, vicious menstrual cramps, irregular periods and ovulation under control. Let's get your body—inside and outside—

in the best shape possible so that you are brimming over with the cleanest, healthiest and most baby-licious blood, nutrients and life-generating essences possible.

Yeah, baby!

OK, I know that not all of you reading this book are like Sarah; you're not looking to get pregnant right now, but most of you, one day, will want to be mothers. For that reason, preparing your Eden of fertility NOW is imperative so that when you want to take the leap into motherhood, your body and mind are raring to go.

"But, Aimee, I'm not even in a serious relationship."

It doesn't matter. You need to get ready now and stay ready because if you're like most women these days, Sarah included, you're waiting until your midthirties to have children, and unfortunately, the closer you get to forty, the more your fertility quotient declines.

What's a fertility quotient? Your fertility quotient is your probability of getting pregnant easily and successfully, carrying a full-term pregnancy and delivering a healthy baby. Bottom line: the older you get, the less likely you are to have a full-term pregnancy that will result in a genetically healthy bambino, because as you age, your baby-making eggs age too and your palace just isn't as proficient as it once was.

In this chapter, I am going to show you the best ways to improve your fertility quotient, work out all your hormonal kinks, get your palace in pristine condition and make your eggs essence-licious. This way, when you want to get pregnant, hopefully it'll be a breeze and you can avoid the tumultuous and exhausting world of fertility treatments. Because, ladies, in case you didn't know, dealing with infertility isn't fun. Besides the obvious emotional turmoil of not being able to have a child when you want one, dealing with infertility involves loads of medical tests and procedures, early-morning doctors' visits, constant monitoring of cervical mucus, timed and unsexy sex and the agonizing, daily stress of wondering if this is the month you'll actually get pregnant.

I'm sure you have at least one girlfriend who has been struggling to get pregnant for over a year or two. I'm sure you know at least one girl who's undergone in vitro fertilization (IVF) treatment. I'm sure you know at least one girl who's taken Clomid (a fertility drug that attempts to induce ovulation). I'm sure you know at least one woman who's had a miscarriage.

It's no wonder. Infertility currently affects about seven million women and their partners in the United States. That's twelve percent of the reproductive-age population.

"Aimee, what exactly is infertility?"

I'm glad you asked. The definition of infertility, according to RESOLVE: The National Infertility Association, is "a disease or condition of the reproductive system often diagnosed after a couple has **one year** of unprotected, **well-timed** intercourse or if the woman suffers from multiple miscarriages [emphasis mine]. Infertility can be male or female related."

Let's break down this definition based on the two most important points; I bolded them for you.

One year. This means twelve months or twelve menstrual cycles, depending on the regularity of your period. This means having unprotected sex for **one year** before you rush to your gynecologist's office and take Clomid. **One year** before you start going crazy on Google, or join the infertility chat rooms and start diagnosing yourself. **One year** to take all the steps I outline in this chapter before you fall into the labyrinthine and very costly, not always successful, emotionally draining and exhausting world of fertility treatments.

Now, I get that sometimes **one year**, especially when you start trying to have a baby at age thirty-five, or thirty-seven, or forty-one, is a long time. I understand that you may want to speed things up. If that's the case, then before you start freaking out that you're not getting pregnant, start applying what I say in this book. Doing so NOW will put your palace in the best shape possible to get pregnant when you decide it's bambino time. Even if you're already struggling with infertility (and as I say this, I am giving you a great big hug) and you are beyond that **one year** of trying, you can still apply what I say here to improve your chances of one day having a healthy baby.

Next there's the business of **well-timed** sex.

Well-timed sex is a huge part of the fertility equation. Well-timed sex means you know when you are ovulating, and you start having unprotected sex (if you wish to get pregnant) three days prior to ovulation. This issue of timing is majorly important because you can get pregnant ONLY when you are ovulating.

What Your Ovulation Should Look Like

Ovulation occurs at the midpoint of a menstrual cycle, so if you have a twenty-eight-day cycle, then you should ovulate around day fourteen (where day one is the first day of your period).

Clues that you are about to ovulate:

- Three or so days before actual ovulation (day ten or eleven in a twenty-eight-day cycle) you should see some cervical

continued

mucus (CM). It should be small in amount (just a pea-sized dollop), moist or sticky and white or cream in color.

- The day before and the day of ovulation (days thirteen and fourteen in a twenty-eight-day cycle) the amount of mucus will significantly increase (about a teaspoon's worth) and it will become very stretchy and egg-whitish looking.
- On the day right after ovulation (day fifteen in a twenty-eight-day cycle) there is a marked change in mucus appearance; the amount diminishes and it gets sticky again. Within a day or two there should be no more mucus.

Ovulation is when one of your ovaries (you have two) drops an egg, and one of your fallopian tubes (you have two) sweeps it up so it can be fertilized by a sperm that happens to be hanging around waiting for some action. So you see, that's why it's important to have sex *before* you ovulate, so that the sperm are ready and waiting for that egg.

How Pregnancy Happens

When you are ovulating normally, your body, every month, drops a mature egg from one of your ovaries (you have two). This egg is then taken up by one of your fallopian tubes (you have two of these too). The fallopian tube, with its fingerlike projections, sweeps the egg up into the tube, where it may meet a ready and waiting sperm. The sperm then fertilizes the egg, creating an embryo. The fallopian tube's fingerlike projections then sweep up the embryo farther into the fallopian tube and eventually into the uterus (each of the fallopian tubes opens right up into the uterus). Once in the uterus, the embryo implants into your lush uterine lining, where it will remain and grow into a baby over the next nine months.

From the time your period begins until ovulation, your ovaries develop several follicles, all of which contain an egg that can be ovulated. Over a period of approximately two weeks, these follicles grow bigger and bigger. At the time of ovulation, certain hormonal interactions cause the largest follicle to rupture an egg that can be fertilized by a sperm and become a baby. The key to remember here is that, of the several follicles that are developing, only the largest, most mature one is ovulated. The whole process is Darwinesque—it's "survival of the fittest"; the egg that is ovulated is the one that is most optimal for creating a healthy baby. The rest of the follicles are subpar and will just die off. Makes sense, doesn't it?

Egg and Sperm Timing

The egg is capable of being fertilized by a sperm for only twelve to twenty-four hours after ovulation.

The sperm, however, is capable of fertilizing an egg anywhere from forty-eight to seventy-two hours after being ejaculated. But keep in mind, the sperm needs anywhere from six to twelve hours to reach the fallopian tubes.

You see, getting pregnant is all about the timing—you have to have sex one or two days before ovulation or immediately after ovulation for a pregnancy to occur.

For most women in their twenties, ovulation isn't an issue, nor is creating that best dang healthy fertile chosen egg. But as we age, unfortunately, both ovulation and the ability to create a good healthy egg become more difficult, because our ovaries and our eggs age just like we do. Sigh.

Ovaries, as they age, become less efficient and may not ovulate every month. And aging eggs make for poor-quality eggs, which make for poor-quality embryos, which unfortunately make it harder to get pregnant, being that our body wants to carry to term only a baby that is going to be genetically healthy. And aging eggs typically have genetic abnormalities. Not to mention that, as we age, the number of eggs we have in our ovarian reserve (we are born with a set amount of eggs) declines. So, for women who are getting married and having children later in life, this whole aging-ovary-and-egg business isn't the best news.

"Aimee, you're depressing me! What do I do?"

Ladies, I've got one word for you: essence.

Chinese Medicine theory states: plentiful essence increases fertility and longevity. CM theory maintains that a woman with ample essence can easily have a healthy baby in her forties.

"Really?!"

Yes! You see, the quality of a woman's eggs, her ovaries and her entire reproductive system are completely and totally dependent upon the abundance of her essence.

Let's recap the two types of essence I talked about in chapter 5:

- Prenatal essence is before-birth essence. This is the foundation from which we are created. This includes not only what some would refer to as our genetics but also the internal embryonic environment we developed in. So if Mom was a smoker who ate nothing but junk and hated her job, we didn't get the best prenatal essence. Alternatively, if she was the happiest, healthiest pregger gal, we had a great embryonic environment and received a nice chunk of prenatal essence. Unfortunately, prenatal essence is completely out of our control—it is what it is.
- Postnatal essence is after-birth essence. This is the health and longevity that we can create by eating and living as naturally as possible. When it comes to creating postnatal essence, the ball is in your court. Postnatal essence is critical and can override potentially negative dispositions that were passed down to us by our folks. Said another way, an abundance of postnatal essence will assure you longevity and the ability to have a healthy baby later in life. Woo hoo!

All right, take a deep breath, and reread the definitions of pre- and postnatal essence one more time. I totally get it if you are confused right now.

You're probably thinking, "Aimee, if you are in fact correct about this pre- and postnatal essence stuff, how come I turned out healthy when my mom smoked during her entire pregnancy with me?" Or maybe you're wondering, "How can some women who are drug addicts have healthy babies and other women who are health conscious and organic have mentally challenged ones?"

All great questions.

It's possible that the drug addict's baby had a kick-ass grandma who passed on some phenomenal prenatal essence to her daughter (who sadly became a drug addict), and it was this phenomenal prenatal essence that overcame the negative lifestyle factors and made a healthy baby. Similarly, we don't definitively know the long-term health of that drug addict's child; we don't know the reproductive capabilities of that child or the genetic predispositions that may one day pose health issues for that child.

Bottom line: the way in which you live your life directly affects the way your body functions and what you will pass on to your unborn children for generations.

Heavy stuff.

Oftentimes there are other factors that are beyond our control. I'm here to educate you on the factors that are within our control. That means optimizing your postnatal essence by making the best possible lifestyle choices NOW.

So, here we go. To make the best-damn-quality eggs, we *need* to focus on postnatal essence; it's the goods. *And* it's the prenatal essence for our future little ones, get it? Postnatal essence is the antiaging elixir that you can cultivate to assure that you have the best-damn-quality healthy-baby-licious-making machinery ever!

Ladies, if you put some time and energy NOW into preparing your palace and making your internal environment as healthy and hospitable as possible, you can and will increase your odds of having a healthy and viable pregnancy in your thirties and forties. Think about it. If someone said to you, "I got this great apartment to let for forty weeks rent free—you want it?" what would run through your head? You'd probably ask some questions like,

What kind of shape is it in?
Is it regularly maintained or is it falling apart?
Is there a place for me to get some good healthy eats nearby?
Is it on a busy street or is it quiet?
Is it cozy?

It's the same for that little person to whom you hope to give birth one day. If your insides aren't in great shape, quiet and peaceful, being nurtured and brimming over with essence, why on earth would someone want to live there?

The Birth Control Pill: My Opinion

Bottom line: chemically suppressing your body's baby-making system—for years, sometimes decades—just doesn't jibe with me. The birth control pill, via synthetic hormones, manipulates your body so that ovulation doesn't occur (that's why women who are on the Pill don't see any cervical mucus or have a sex drive).

For some women in their thirties who went on the Pill at the age of sixteen or so, this system shutdown has been going for nearly fifteen years! You tell me, how efficient do you think a system that's been shut down for fifteen years would run when it's suddenly expected to do so again? Personally, I think it'd be a bit rusty. Don't you?

Of course I recognize the important role the Pill plays in preventing unwanted pregnancies. However, I feel it's unsound practice to put a young woman on the Pill because of menstrual cramps

continued

or migraines or acne or mood swings or polycystic ovaries or any other symptom for that matter, as this does not directly deal with her root issue. Rather, it just shuts down an intricate hormonal system for however long, to the possible detriment of her fertility quotient.

Ladies, here's some science for you to ponder: a study published in *Gynecological Endocrinology* showed that women who had just stopped taking the Pill had "major" cycle disturbances (like irregular ovulation and periods) in comparison with women who never took the Pill. This report also showed that it took up to nine months for women with a history of taking the Pill to establish a regular menstrual cycle after discontinuing the Pill. Another study published by the esteemed journal *Fertility and Sterility* showed that women who took the Pill for more than two years had a greater incidence of miscarriage. Yikes!

Now, before we get down to the essence of the business—yes, that cheesy pun was intentional—I'm going to add another layer to the timing matter: **regular menstruation**.

Ladies, regular menstruation is imperative for timely ovulation. If you are not menstruating regularly, chances are you are not ovulating regularly, and *boy, oh boy*, does that make getting pregnant difficult.

Statistics show that one of the most common reasons for female infertility is an ovulation disorder. An ovulation disorder means a woman may be menstruating, but she's ovulating either too early, too late or not at all, or she's ovulating poor-quality, nonfertilizable eggs.

What Your Period Should Be Like

- It should come regularly every month without fail.
- Periods should be between twenty-eight and thirty-two days apart (where the first day of bleeding, not spotting, is counted as day one of your cycle).

continued

- It should come on quietly, with slight breast tenderness and very little cramping.
- It is normal for some women to experience a touch of spotting the day before their actual period begins. It is not normal to experience spotting for a few days or a week before your period begins.
- Your period should last four to six days; it should start heavier on days one and two (about eight tablespoons of blood each day or soaking a super tampon every three to four hours), slowly tapering off the last few days (anywhere between two and six tablespoons of blood each day or soaking a regular tampon every three to four hours).
- Bleeding should not at any point be excessive, meaning you should not leak through a super tampon in two hours.
- On the other end of the spectrum, if you need to wear only pantie liners when you have your period, even on day one or two, that's not normal.
- The blood should be a garnetlike fresh red color; it shouldn't be dark brown or pale pink.
- Small, wet-Kleenex-tissue-like, dime-sized clots are considered normal; big quarter-sized ones are not.

Tell me:

Is your period regular?
Are you ovulating each month?

If your answer to either question is a pause followed by "I don't know," then you need to start tracking both your monthly period and your signs of ovulation so you can figure out exactly what's going on with your body.

"How? This sounds like work!"

Aw, c'mon, it's easy. All this is going to require is a pen, a calendar and a little self-observation.

Tracy came to me eager to prepare for her third IVF cycle. She was thirty-seven, and after her last two IVFs her doctors told her she had "poor-quality eggs" (grade 1 and 2 eggs, on a scale of 0—4, where 4 is the best quality). And with each cycle she produced only seven follicles (five eggs fertilized on the first cycle and only three eggs fertilized on the second cycle). She was interested in acupuncture because she read that it can improve the success rate of IVF by thirty to forty percent.

We had three months until her next IVF cycle. So I quickly got down to business: I put her on a clean, organic and nondead diet, got her exercising four days a week (she'd gained fifteen pounds from the hormones she took during her previous IVFs), gave her an individualized Chinese herbal regimen, cod-liver oil and spirulina and encouraged her to come for acupuncture once a week. She also began doing some of the "Perking Up the Palace" recommendations in this chapter.

In three months, her menstrual cycle changed. On her new CM regimen, her periods, once very heavy, crampy and clotty, were lighter, clot free and cramp free—and she had little to no PMS.

When it came time for her next IVF, she produced thirteen follicles (that's almost twice as many as she produced during her previous IVFs); of nine eggs fertilized, three were grade 4, five were grade 3 and one was grade 2.

As I write this, Tracy is twenty weeks pregnant!

Put a number one on your calendar the first day of bleeding; this is day one of your menstrual cycle (if you spot before your period begins, note this with "sp," but do not count it as the first day of your menstruation). Then mark on your calendar when you start to see cervical mucus (CM). For a small pea-sized amount of moist mucus just write "CM"; when it starts to get more copious (say, a teaspoon or two) and egg-whitish, write "EW." That's it. These little markings on your calendar will help you figure out if your menstrual cycle is regular and whether you are actually ovulating.

"But what if my cycle isn't regular, Aimee?"
"What if I have debilitating cramps with my period?"
"What if my boobs KILL me before my period?"
"What if I don't see any vaginal discharge EVER?"
"What if I see vaginal discharge all the time?"
All shall be revealed.

· REPAIRING THE PALACE ·

Chinese Medicine views regular monthly menstruation, ovulation and overall reproductive health as a function of one's essence. Of course, the circulation of Qi and blood plays a very important role in keeping your palace running smoothly, but without an adequate amount of essence, your Qi and blood have no energy to keep your palace functioning properly. When this happens, the palace is in disarray and so are you. How will you know things have gone awry? You'll have raging PMS, hormonally related headaches and acne, an irregular period and erratic ovulations. So, first things first, in order to repair your palace, we need to get your Qi, blood and essence in check.

Quick Fixes for Menstrual Cramps

Drink turmeric tea or red raspberry leaf tea. Add cinnamon to either. Drink up to three times per day when you have bad cramps.

Massage ginger oil on your lower abdomen, then put on a hot-water bottle and let the heat and the ginger soothe your cramps. You can do this several times per day to relieve your cramping.

Acupressure: find the sore spot on the inside of your lower leg about 4 fingers' width above your inner ankle bone; this is the acupuncture point Spleen 6 and it is great at relieving

continued

---

menstrual cramps. Gently massage this spot on both legs for 2 minutes. You can do this a few times per day to relieve cramps. Beware: don't do this if you are or could be pregnant, as this point can induce labor!

I know, and here you just wanted to get rid of your PMS!

Girl, most of the time it's your lifestyle that causes PMS and other hormonally related issues. The way you manage stress, the amount of exercise you get and what you eat positively or negatively affect the way your Qi and blood circulate. And the efficient circulation—or not—of Qi and blood and the amount of essence you have directly affect your fertility quotient and overall reproductive health. Get it? Other times there are structural issues in your reproductive organs (like endometriosis or scar tissue from a previous surgery) that block the flow of Qi and blood regardless of how much essence you have. These structural issues need to be investigated by a reproductive endocrinologist (RE) and usually require medical intervention in conjunction with lifestyle changes to get your body into the best baby-making health possible. But since I'm neither a surgeon nor a reproductive endocrinologist, I'm going to focus on teaching you how to manage the lifestyle stressors that are negatively affecting your essence, Qi, blood and reproductive health and causing you hormonal distress.

Below are the six main factors that you need to get a handle on. One or more of them may be causing your erratic-bitch-from-hell-bloated-painful-boobs menstrual cycle and preventing you from having an optimal fertility quotient.

1. **STRESS.** I know, I know, I'm like a broken record! But, ladies, stress is probably the number one culprit that burns up your essence, stops up your Qi and gives you horrible menstrual cramps. Chronic stress ravages your body and leaves you with a nil fertility quotient and major hormonal imbalances.

We talked about this in chapter 3, but let me go over it again. Ultimately, the stress response is in place to protect and support us when we are faced with a threat through the release of two key hormones: cortisol and adrenaline. The release of these chemicals causes a cascade of reactions in our body: our heart rate increases, our blood vessels constrict to prevent blood loss in case of injury, our pupils dilate so we can see better, and our blood sugar ramps up, giving us an energy boost to either fight or flee. In reaction to this chemical cascade, our bodies go into automatic overdrive, enabling us to move and think faster, hit harder, see better, hear more acutely and jump higher for a short burst of time. So, in actuality, stress and the hormones associated with it are healthy and even protective when activated in MODERATION or in response to a real threat.

However, in today's world, stress is by no means moderate or rare. This is where the essence-robbing problems arise. You see, the more the stress cascade is activated (say, every time you see your boss, talk to your mother or worry about whether the person you're crushing on will call), the harder it is to shut off. Instead of the body chilling out once a crisis has passed, your stress hormones, heart rate and blood pressure remain elevated because the body hasn't had ample time to filter out the excess adrenaline and cortisol. This excess of adrenaline and cortisol negatively affects the way your body normally regulates its other hormones, and this, ladies, really takes a toll on your essence and reproductive system! These excess stress hormones will cause things like raging PMS, irregular and painful periods, weight gain, pimples, cellulite and erratic ovulation. Seriously!

All of us could use ways to better manage our stress. Go back and really, truly incorporate into your daily life the tools I offer you in chapter 3. Get a handle on your stress, CTFO daily, amass more essence, improve your fertility quotient and manage that annoying PMS! You can do it!

2. **ANXIETY AND DEPRESSION.** Repeated episodes of anxiety and depression have the same effects on the body as the stress cascade. The bottom line is that anxiety and depression produce a plethora of those same stress hormones (cortisol and adrenaline). To recap, these hormones will deprive your body of baby-making essence, affect the circulation of Qi and blood and make your period and ovulation irregular. Not good.

Do you feel like you struggle with anxiety and depression?

Can you tell if these emotions are causing you to be a hormonal mess?

Do you see that your moods affect your period whether it's horrible PMS, debilitating cramps, acne, killer bloat or sore breasts?

Do you experience big emotional highs and lows around your period?

If so, go back and reread chapter 4 and apply the tools I recommend there. Also, you might seriously consider speaking with a psychotherapist about what's making you feel anxious or what's making you feel desperately sad all the time. Honestly, it'll help you emotionally and physically.

3. **WEIGHT.** This is a big culprit when it comes to a dysfunctional female reproductive system, as fat cells store estrogen, and estrogen is a majorly important hormone in an efficient female reproductive system (the other important hormone is progesterone). So if you have too little or too much fat, it will completely disrupt your estrogen levels and this, darlin', is going to completely screw up your ability to menstruate and ovulate regularly.

- **UNDERWEIGHT.** When the body doesn't have enough fat on it, it goes into what I like to call "survival mode." A body in survival mode runs on fear. It doesn't know where its next meal is coming from and it's afraid that it doesn't have enough energy (your body stores energy in fat) to survive a crisis like fighting off a cold or sustaining an injury. Girl, the last thing a body in "survival mode" feels it's capable of doing is getting pregnant and carrying a baby to term. Also, a woman who has a very low percentage of body fat doesn't have enough estrogen to generate a regular menstrual cycle, let alone get pregnant. In fact most underweight women have either very light and infrequent periods or no periods at all. Ladies, the point I'm trying to drive home is, a body with too little fat on it does not have enough essence to sustain a healthy pregnancy, let alone a normal menstrual cycle. If you wanna have a baby, you gotta gain some weight.

- **OVERWEIGHT.** On the other side of the coin, a body with excess weight has excess estrogen (as estrogen is stored in fat cells), which disrupts the body's ability to carry out a normal menstruation and ovulation. Excess estrogen also predisposes women to illnesses like endometriosis, ovarian cysts, breast cancer and uterine fibroids—all of which will really hinder one's chances of becoming preggers! Not to mention, a body carrying around excess weight has to work extra hard to do simple things like move, digest food and circulate blood; it definitely isn't in ideal shape to sustain a normal menstrual cycle, let alone a pregnancy.

The best way to decide if your weight is in check is to determine your body mass index (BMI). This is real easy. The formula for determining your BMI is this: (weight $\div$ height^2) $\times$ 703 (using pounds and inches). For example, if you weigh 150 pounds and are 5 feet 5 (65 inches), the calculation would be as follows: $(150 \div 65^2) \times 703 = 24.96$. Get it? Here's a BMI chart so that you can determine what your BMI means:

- **BELOW 18.5.** You're underweight and need to put on some weight to optimize your fertility quotient. Sometimes you just need to gain five pounds. Remember you need some fat in order to sustain healthy bodily functions; without enough body fat, you have no energy to create postnatal essence. Incorporate at least three servings per day of foods with natural, rich fats like olive oil, avocados, nuts, eggs and animal protein (like red meat and chicken) into your diet.

- **18.5–24.9.** You're in the normal BMI range and your weight is optimal for your getting pregnant. However, weight is just one factor that affects your fertility quotient.

- **25.0–29.9.** You're a little overweight and should lose some weight to optimize your fertility quotient. Sometimes even losing five pounds can make a huge difference in your ability to get pregnant.

- **30.0 OR ABOVE.** If you fall into this BMI range, you fall under the medical definition of "obese" (which is twenty or more pounds overweight). I'd recommend you get on board with an exercise regimen and follow the nutritional advice at the end of this chapter in conjunction with the information in chapters 5 and 6. Make it a serious goal to drop some weight. Your body and your reproductive system will thank you.

4. **DIET.** I know what you're thinking: "Aimee and her obsession with diet!" Yes, now you're getting it. You are what you eat! If you don't eat a good clean, organic, unprocessed diet, your body and all its essence, Qi and blood will suffer and so will you with terrible PMS, irritability, and a whacked-out reproductive system. To optimize your fertility quotient, apply everything in chapters 5 and 6. In addition, at the end of this chapter are my favorite hormone-balancing foods—if you're serious about getting your hormones in order and repairing your palace, incorporate these foods into your diet.

5. **EXERCISE.** Too much or too little exercise can really affect your fertility quotient. However, exercise, like weight, is a hard issue to make definitive recommendations about, as everyone's body is so entirely different. My general rule of thumb is four to five days a week of at least thirty minutes of exercise. The level of intensity depends upon your comfort level and your goals. If you have a high BMI and are looking to lose weight to optimize your fertility quotient, then some heart-pounding, sweat-soaking workouts may be what you need. On the other hand if you are a long-distance runner and need to put on some weight to increase your fertility quotient, then I recommend you adopt some less-intense means of exercise like restorative yoga or walking (and eat some healthy fatty foods). Bottom line: exercise is imperative for optimal health, but like everything else, you must find a balance with it. Too much or too little of anything isn't good for you.

6. **PHYSICAL ILLNESS.** One of the most common illnesses that affect women's ability to reproduce is a thyroid disorder. Either an overactive or underactive thyroid will disrupt your menstrual cycle and your body's ability to ovulate regularly. This is because the body is either functioning like it's on speed (hyperthyroidism) or functioning too slowly (hypothyroidism). Either one of these illnesses can affect your fertility quotient and make it very hard for your body to generate an ample amount of essence. If you suspect you have a thyroid disorder, request a referral to an endocrinologist from your primary care doc.

One thing to keep in mind is that a lot of times your thyroid may not be functioning optimally but this dysfunction may not show up on lab tests. Following a clean diet, getting enough sleep and exercising can help bring your body back into balance. Also, even subclinical thyroid disorders respond very positively to acupuncture and Chinese herbs. Go to Nccaom.org to find a qualified practitioner in your area. There are also other physical illnesses that will affect a woman's essence and fertility quotient, like cancer, multiple sclerosis and diabetes. The bottom line is that you need to amp up your postnatal essence so that your body can manage the illness and get its reproductive system back on track. When you're dealing with chronic illness, it's important to employ every essence-building opportunity available to get your health back in tip-top shape.

Potential Symptoms of an Overactive Thyroid (Hyperthyroidism)

- Nervousness, anxiety and irritability
- Weight loss
- Fast and/or irregular heart rate
- Feeling hot all the time
- Excessive perspiration
- Ravenous appetite
- Restless sleep and insomnia
- Muscle weakness
- Trembling hands
- More-frequent bowel movements
- Shorter and scantier menstrual flow
- Bulging eyes
- Goiter (enlarged thyroid gland)

Potential Symptoms of an Underactive Thyroid (Hypothyroidism)

- Fatigue
- Depression
- Feeling too cold
- Weight gain
- Dry or itchy skin
- Thin, dry hair or hair loss
- Puffy face, hands and feet
- Decreased taste and smell
- Constipation
- Poor memory and concentration
- Hoarse voice
- Irregular or heavy menstruation
- Infertility
- High cholesterol

· PERKING UP THE PALACE ·

All right, now that you understand the six major lifestyle factors that you need to address to repair your palace, create abundant essence and improve your fertility quotient, let's talk about some more-specific fertility-enhancing tools you can incorporate into your life easily and almost without effort. Seriously!

EATING YOUR WAY TO HORMONAL BLISS

As you know by now, I'm a HUGE fan of a great diet! If you are hormonally challenged—you experience erratic menstrual cycles, horrible cramps, raging PMS or hormonally related acne or weight gain; you're having a hard time getting pregnant or you've been diagnosed with endometriosis or polycystic ovarian syndrome—these CM-inspired dietary recommendations are for YOU! Even if you're just looking to improve your fertility quotient, incorporating these dietary suggestions will be to your advantage.

The specific foods I have listed here have essence-building, hormone-balancing and inflammation-reducing effects. Combine this dietary advice with the advice I give in chapters 5 and 6 and you will power up your postnatal essence, regulate your reproductive system and dramatically improve your fertility quotient. Just do it!

1. Eat lean animal protein and monounsaturated and polyunsaturated oils! These foods are rich in hormone-balancing essential fatty acids, which make them great for improving your essence and fertility quotient. However, when it comes to balancing your hormones, I am going to recommend that you get your protein more from fish, nuts and beans than animal meats. Of course, I still recommend you eat animal meats, but when you do, remember to ALWAYS eat veggies, as they balance each other.

   "Veggies balance meats? Why?"

Generally speaking, animal protein is very acidic. Acidic foods exacerbate inflammation in your body; they can make your liver toxic if you overdo it (or don't balance them with alkalinizing foods) and your PMS worse. So the key here is NOT to avoid eating animal meat; it's to be sure you eat alkalinizing veggies and fruit to balance out the acidity of the animal protein. Girl, it's all about balance, you know that. Eat alkalinizing veggies and fruits in conjunction with acidic animal protein, and you'll keep your hormones in balance and painful-period, sore-breasted and acne-causing inflammation at bay. Get it?

Keep in Mind

A serving size is
  - for meat, fish or poultry, the size of your palm.
  - for rice or pasta, the size of a tennis ball.

- Organic eggs: consume four to six per week with the yolk (note that this recommendation is slightly different from the six to eight eggs/week I recommended in chapter 6). Soft-boil, hard-boil or panfry using organic butter, ghee or coconut or sesame oil.
- Deep-sea, cold-water fish: consume six to eight servings a week of safe deep-sea, cold-water fish, such as salmon, sardines, mackerel and cod. See the "Something Smells Fishy" section in chapter 6 for more information on which fish are safe to eat. Broil, steam or grill using organic olive, sesame or coconut oil.
- Free-range, hormone- and antibiotic-free poultry: consume two to four servings a week. Grill, bake or cook on your stove top using organic olive, sesame or coconut oil.

- Free-range, hormone- and antibiotic-free red meat: consume two to four servings a week of lean meat such as lamb, venison, grass-fed beef, buffalo and pork. Eat as lean as possible. Grass-fed beef is ideal. Pan-sear, grill or broil. Using an oil or butter with meats is not necessary, as these meats contain a good amount of fat all on their own. If you're afraid of the meat sticking to your cookware, use a smidgen of organic coconut or sesame oil, butter or ghee.

- Organic, hormone- and antibiotic-free dairy: intake should be very limited or avoided altogether. Organic nonhomogenized yogurt (such as Stonyfield Farm) is OK to have once or twice a week. Remember, yogurt is fermented and easier to digest. In general, goat-milk and sheep-milk products are better choices than cow-milk products, because they tend to be less allergenic and inflammatory. Try some sheep's milk yogurt in a smoothie or for a calcium-boosting treat—you might just love it!

- Organic seeds and nuts: two to four tablespoons per day. Nuts and seeds, such as flaxseeds (grind them yourself, and do not use flaxseed oil [see box on next page]), almonds, cashews, walnuts, Brazil nuts, filberts, sunflower seeds, sesame seeds and pumpkin seeds, are a great source of energy during the day. Did you notice I didn't mention peanuts? If you're going to have peanuts, they MUST be organic, as not only are peanuts very allergenic and inflammatory, but nonorganic peanuts also contain the cancer-causing agent called aflatoxin. And that's just no good for your health.

- Organic oils: olive, coconut and sesame are all great for you and rich in essential fatty acids. Cook with them (keeping in mind what I've said about cooking with olive oil back in chapter 6) or put them on your salads. Try to get in one tablespoon per day of one of these oils.

The Thing About Flax Seed Oil

The only way to get health benefits from flax seeds is to eat the ground seed. Taking flax seed in oil form unfortunately does not offer us all the health benefits of flax.

You see, flax seed oil is a very sensitive and unstable oil, and at even slightly high temperatures (like that of our body—98.6 degrees Fahreheit), it can go rancid, offering us no nutritional value and potential harm. Just eat ground flax seed!

2. Eat LOADS of organic veggies! You should have one serving of a veggie with each meal and ALWAYS eat veggies when you have animal protein, as they balance each other (to recap: animal protein is acidic and veggies are alkaline—eating them together keeps your hormones in balance and painful-period, sore-breasted and acne-causing inflammation at bay). Eat as many colors of veggies as possible. Green veggies are particularly good at cleansing the liver, regulating PMS and clearing up your skin.

Prepare these veggies by steaming, sautéing or roasting them in organic olive oil, coconut oil or canola oil. Be sure to cook your veggies al dente, as overcooked veggies lose most of their nutrients. A vegetable cooked properly should have a bit of bite to it.

- Leafy greens: lettuce, spinach, kale, chard, collards, watercress and kelp
- Cruciferous veggies: broccoli, Brussels sprouts, cabbage, cauliflower and bok choy
- Onion and garlic. These two are a great source of anti-aging antioxidants. Eat 'em often.
- Root veggies: carrots, beets, jicama, daikon, radish, rutabagas, turnips and parsnips. These veggies are rich in essence-boosting antioxidants, fiber and nutrients

(like folic acid and beta-carotene) that help balance our hormones.

- Medicinal mushrooms: maitake, shiitake, reishi (aka ganoderma lucidum or *ling zhi*), and wood ear (aka black mushrooms). These mushrooms have been a part of the CM healing tradition since AD 200. These medicinal mushrooms are used to enhance the immune system, fight off cancer and boost postnatal essence. Many cancer specialists have taken to recommending medicinal mushrooms to their patients, as many scientists, particularly those at Cancer Research UK, have found evidence that these foods actually do have immunity-enhancing and anticancer properties.

- Legumes: lentils, split peas, and beans, including garbanzo, pinto and lima beans. These foods are loaded with healthy, banana-like-bowel-movement-promoting fiber and minerals like magnesium that help ease menstrual cramps.

- Sweet potatoes and yams: these guys are loaded with antioxidants and hormone-balancing vitamins. Eat at least one per week. To reduce the sugar load of these starchy veggies, be sure to eat them with a good fat, such as olive oil or organic butter.

Eat Leafy Green and Cruciferous Veggies Like They're Going out of Style!

Leafy greens and cruciferous vegetables contain a substance called indole-3-carbinol (I3C), which has been shown to block the production of toxic estrogens that cause diseases like endometriosis, fibrocystic breasts, breast cancer, ovarian cancer, uterine cancer and cervical dysplasia. From a CM standpoint, these veggies help keep your liver Qi moving—and a woman with free-flowing liver Qi doesn't have PMS!

3. **WHOLE GRAINS:** it's imperative that you eat only whole grains, as they are high in fiber, are loaded with naturally occurring vitamins and nutrients and have a lower sugar load than refined grains. All these whole-grain characteristics make them ideal for helping keep your liver detoxed, your hormones balanced and your colon clean!

- Alkaline nongluten grains: wild rice, brown rice, brown basmati rice, brown jasmine rice, millet, buckwheat, amaranth and quinoa. These are the healthiest grains out there. Eat one to two servings per day. Avoid—at all costs—white rice; it offers you zilch for nutrition.
- Acidic gluten grains: wheat, rye and barley. These acidic grains increase estrogen levels, inhibit proper liver function, are highly allergenic (read box) and make your body phlegmy. Try your best to avoid these altogether. A serving or two of organic stone-ground, whole wheat bread is acceptable once in a while. Hey, everything in moderation, right?

The Weigh-in on Wheat

Stone-ground organic whole wheat is good for you. But here's the thing: wheat isn't as rich in age-fighting, essence-boosting antioxidants as other whole grains. And wheat is notoriously difficult to digest. Many people have a sensitivity to wheat proteins and don't even realize it.

Do you feel bloated, crampy or gassy or have diarrhea after eating bread or pasta or soy sauce? You may be wheat intolerant.

Wheat also contains a protein called gluten that many people have a genetic inability to digest properly. The genetic autoimmune disorder is called celiac disease (CD).

CD affects 1 in every 133 Americans. If you think you have gluten sensitivity, the only way you can really tell is to cut wheat

continued

out of your diet and monitor your symptoms. If you suspect that you have an inability to digest wheat or someone in your family has been diagnosed with CD (thus raising the probability that you have it as well), see a board-certified gastroenterologist to definitively rule out celiac disease.

Keep in mind, you may have a gluten sensitivity and not test positive for CD.

Here are some good Web sites for more information: aafa.org, and celiacdiseasecenter.columbia.edu.

- Oats: consume only in the form of organic steel-cut oatmeal. You can have oatmeal three times per week. No instant oatmeal and definitely NO flavored, prepackaged oatmeal.
- Corn: limit to fresh organic corn. Have corn on the cob or cooked corn as a side dish two to three times per week. When I recommend corn, I am mainly recommending fresh organic corn. Many processed and packaged foods contain corn, but it's usually the genetically modified (GM) kind, as corn is one of the top GM foods in the U.S. (right next to soy). So if you're buying a product made from corn, be sure to read labels and avoid GM corn and anything containing high-fructose corn syrup, because it is toxic and B-A-D for you! For safe measures on avoiding all GM foods, go back to chapter 6 and reread the "Beware of Clones" section.
- A word on spelt. Spelt does contain gluten—the same difficult-to-digest protein that's found in wheat—which makes it more acidic; however, it contains less gluten than traditional wheat breads. OK to have two times per week, as spelt is relatively acidic (but not as acidic as wheat, rye and barley) and can increase estrogen levels

and inhibit proper liver function. Again, everything in moderation.

- Cereals, breads, pastas, rice cakes, crackers, pancakes, muffins and popcorn should all be organic, whole grain, made with natural ingredients and consumed only one to two times per week. Rice-based breads and pastas are your best choice. Always consume these foods with good fats, such as organic nut butters, organic butter, ghee, olive oil or coconut oil, to reduce their sugar load.

4. **FRUITS AND JUICES:** again remember, any food with a high sugar content, even if it's natural sugar, should be eaten in moderation, as a high sugar load increases insulin resistance and thereby increases hormonal imbalances and inflammation.

- Fruits with the least sugar: melons, berries, grapefruit and avocado (yes, it's a fruit!). Consume four to eight servings per week.
- Moderate- to high-sugared fruits: apples, pears, plums, peaches, citrus, bananas and figs. Consume two to four servings per week.
- Dried fruits are very high in sugar and should not be consumed at all.
- One hundred percent pure juices, NOT from concentrate. You can have four fluid ounces per day of pure cranberry or pomegranate juice, as these two fruit juices are great for cleansing the liver. Because they are so tart, it is smart to dilute these juices with water: one-third juice to two-thirds water.

5. **SWEETENERS.** Let's face it, we all have a sweet tooth once in a while. . . . Healthy organic sweeteners can be consumed very moderately: maple syrup, molasses, malt syrup, raw honey, raw agave nectar, stevia, rice syrup and sorghum syrup.

6. OTHER FOODSTUFFS

- Alcohol: limit. Studies show that consuming five drinks per week increases the risk of breast cancer. Avoid wine, as the yeast and sugar content is very high and will exacerbate any existing hormonal imbalances. If you are not pregnant and want a drink, have purified alcohols such as top-shelf vodkas, scotches, whiskeys and gins. Read the "Vodka Rocks!" section in chapter 6. Bottom line: avoid alcohol if you think you could be pregnant or are actively trying to get pregnant.
- Caffeine: coffee or tea should always be organic. Limit yourself to one cup of organic tea or coffee a day. Avoid if you think you could be pregnant or are actively trying to get pregnant.

What to Avoid When Trying to Get Pregnant

alcohol	pesticides
caffeine	aspartame
cigarettes	plastics
canned foods	processed lunch meats
sugar (decrease)	processed foods, especially
cheese/milk (decrease)	those containing toxic soy
food additives	derivatives hormonally treated
cosmetic chemicals	meats/foods tofu
MSG	

And, ladies, remember from chapter 5, the Big Four phlegm-producing foods that we need to steer clear of:

- Sugar
- Soy
- White flour
- Dairy (in moderation, as indicated in chapter 5)

1. Meditation for Preparing Your Palace

Perform this exercise daily, from day one of your period until ovulation.

Step 1. Lie down on your back, with your eyes closed. CTFO and breathe deeply. Notice any areas of tension you feel in your body from your head to your neck, down your arms and hands, through your torso, down your abdomen, buttocks, thighs, calves and feet. Tense the tight areas in your body even more, one by one. Breathe in, inhaling deeply down into your lower abdomen. Push your stomach out as you breathe in. Each inhalation should be five seconds; hold it for two seconds and then exhale for another five seconds. With each exhalation, breathe out the tension in your body.

Focus your attention on the tension, the breath and the relaxation. Nothing more. When the tension in that particular part of your body is gone, move on to the next part. When you feel relaxed throughout your body, and your mind is clear, begin the visualization below, continuing the deep-breathing exercise, breathing deep into your abdomen and relaxing with each exhalation.

Step 2. Now focus your breath down into your pelvis, breathing into your uterus. Let the uterus draw the breath in itself. Let these breaths be cleansing. The uterus has one energetic function. It is downward. It takes the blood and the breath in through the top and lets them out downward through the bottom. Think of the uterus as a receptive, essence-filled organ. It draws in blood and energy through the breath to prepare a gardenlike home for a baby. Picture a lush, receptive and welcoming garden when you picture your uterus. With every breath in, you bring clean and beautiful energy in through the top of the uterus. With every exhalation, breathe out any impurities downward through the bottom of the uterus. Any pain, any toxins, any impurities, are released downward, with each breath. You are helping to prepare your luxurious palace for implantation. This is a pure, flourishing, abundant home. It is open, receptive and fertile. It cannot afford to have any toxins. Release them. When your uterus feels pure, open and receptive, you are finished.

2. MEDITATION FOR BABY-MAKING NIRVANA

Step 1. Repeat step one from the above meditation for preparing your palace.

Step 2. Breathe in very deeply, and concentrate on bringing your breath from your nose, down the midline of your body, between your breasts and down your abdomen, eventually focusing your breath down to your uterus. Let the breath energy pool here.

Breathe in cleansing, purifying breaths to the uterus and then down to the perineal muscles (the muscles down there). Perform a Kegel exercise (see box on following page). This should be a smooth, continuous movement, with cleansing breaths inward. Concentrate on the uterine lining. It is pure, lush and fertile. It is receptive. Each breath brings fresh, clear energy into the uterus, reviving it with healthy, fertile lining. When you release the Kegel, begin exhalation.

During exhalation, turn the focus of your attention from the uterus back to the tip of your tailbone, then up the spine to the top of your head. Your concentration now is on the upward movement, ending with the midline of the head and out the nose. Repeat from the beginning of step 2 with each inhalation, until there's one smooth, continuous movement.

Getting Down with the "Kegel"

Kegel exercises are for strengthening the muscles around your vagina, uterus and bladder. They're also good for having a better orgasm!

Sign me up—how do I do them?

First, you've got to "Kegel" the correct muscle. To figure out the right muscle, pretend you are urinating and then deliberately stop the flow of urine.

Then, isolate the muscle. While doing the Kegel, be sure to keep your back, abdominal and thigh muscles relaxed so that you can isolate and concentrate more energy into the pelvic-floor muscles you are trying to strengthen.

"Kegel" away while lying or sitting with your knees together: squeeze your "Kegel" muscle and hold the squeeze for ten seconds. Then relax the muscle for a few seconds. Do this ten to twenty times in a row. Work up to three sessions a day. Don't hold your breath during the exercise. Breathe slowly and deeply throughout each repetition.

SOME LIKE IT HOT

Ladies, one thing you must try not to lose sight of is, sex rocks! Sex is a beautiful experience shared by two individuals, and it should be amazing. Unfortunately, it can also begin to lose its luster if all you're focused on is whether this time you're going to get pregnant. Try to keep it hot and heavy. Do whatever you gotta do to keep you and your partner physically, chemically and emotionally engaged in the act of sex. Don't use sex merely as a baby-making mechanism but as a way to connect to your partner.

And—this is huge—don't forget to orgasm! Yes, you heard me. When you have an orgasm, hormones are released and muscles contract that help facilitate the sperm and the egg meeting and mating. Girl, be sure to get off!

SUPPLEMENTS TO SUPPORT THE PALACE

To recap what I said in chapter 6: I'm not a huge fan of vitamin supplementation, as I feel most of our nutrients should come from a clean, healthy and organic diet. However, even I recognize that sometimes we need to pop some pills to help our bodies function better. The first three supplement recommendations for improving your fertility quotient are the same three supplements that I recommended back in chapter 6 (go back and reread about them on pages 133–35). These supplements, I feel, are imperative to achieving optimal health. And when you have optimal health—you have an optimal fertility quotient.

1. Cod Liver Oil
2. Spirulina
3. Probiotics
4. Folic acid: if you are actively trying to get pregnant, you should be getting between six hundred and eight hundred micrograms of folic acid per day. So get yourself on a multivitamin that offers you sufficient folic acid.

My favorite brands:

- **In stores**—Garden of Life Vitamin Code, women's formula
- **Online**—NutriHarmony multivitamin

OTHER BEST BETS TO PERK UP YOUR PALACE

- **DON'T BOTHER ME, I'M SUNNIN'.** Each day, before noon, get two ten-minute doses of direct sunshine, without sunglasses. Sunlight stimulates the pituitary and hypothalamus, responsible for fertility hormones.
- **A HULA-VA FERTILITY QUOTIENT.** Each day do three minutes of hip rotations like hula hoop—it helps to open up the pelvic area and create more blood flow to the uterus.

- **TOUCH ME, BABY.** Do some lower-abdominal self-massage prior to ovulation. Standing up or sitting on a chair, take your pointer and middle fingers and find your hip bones—they are the bony protrusions located about three inches below and four inches lateral to your belly button. Now bend over and press your two fingers deeply into the fleshy pelvic area right next to the hip bones. Hold the position for ten seconds, twice per day. This will help increase blood flow to your ovaries. Do this exercise only on days one through nine of your menstrual cycle.
- **KEEP ME WARM, BABY.** Keep your lower abdomen and feet warm. Use a heating pad or a hot-water bottle on your lower abdomen nightly and keep socks on your feet. Doing these two things will keep the energy of your palace and your kidneys warm and cozy.
- **KEGEL IT, BABY.** Do daily Kegel exercises to strengthen your pelvic cavity and the muscles surrounding your vagina, bladder and uterus.

ACUPUNCTURE AND CHINESE HERBS FOR YOUR PALACE

Being a practitioner of Chinese Medicine, I have to say something about the usefulness of both acupuncture and Chinese herbs in regulating a woman's menstrual cycle and improving her fertility quotient. Both acupuncture and Chinese herbs have been used for centuries to improve blood flow and circulation to a woman's palace.

It has been scientifically proven that by inserting tiny needles in specific areas of your body, acupuncture improves uterine blood flow and ovulation, regulates menstrual cycles and curbs PMS. Several articles have been published in scientific journals like *Fertility and Sterility, Human Reproduction* and *Gynecological and Obstetric Investigation* on the effects of acupuncture on women's menstrual cycles, their endocrine system and the success of fertility treatments. To sum up the research, scientists have found that acupuncture can help with

- regulating the menstrual cycle
- regulating and inducing ovulation
- balancing the endocrine (hormonal) system
- improving the blood flow to the pelvic cavity, specifically the uterus
- increasing the chance of pregnancy for women undergoing in vitro fertilization (IVF).

And for your man, it has been shown to

- invigorate and revitalize aged sperm.
- enhance sperm count and motility (the way sperm move).

Specific Chinese herbal formulations are also used in repairing and preparing your palace. Depending on your specific presentation, a board-certified Chinese herbalist can make you your own special fertility-quotient-enhancing concoction. Chinese herbs are prescribed according to specific herbal properties such as acupuncture meridian entered, functions, clinical use, major combinations and dosage. Don't worry if it sounds complicated; board-certified Chinese herbalists are up on the current pharmacological research on Chinese herbs, including their potential drug interactions; antimicrobial, antiviral and antifungal effects; and effects on blood pressure, smooth muscle, hormones, the central nervous system and gynecology.

Word to the wise: go to only a qualified and NCCAOM-board-certified acupuncturist and herbalist for treatment (go to nccaom.org to find a qualified practitioner in your area). Unfortunately there are practitioners out there who are not as qualified to treat you as they should be. Be smart and check out the credentials of any and all medical professionals you seek the advice of. And DO NOT self-treat with Chinese herbs; just because they are natural, they are not always safe.

All right, ladies, now you are geared up to go out and make your palace pristine! Yeah, baby! Next, we're going to work on your beauty from the inside out!

8

Beauty you can't Buy at sephora

CROW'S-FEET, DRY skin, drooping eyelids, neck wattles, eyebrow furrows, brown spots—you name it, they all SUCK!

But you know what sucks even more? That's life. For all of us. Girls, we are going to get old and envy younger versions of ourselves. We have no choice about aging, but we certainly don't have to rush it along by indulging in bad habits. Instead, let's choose to age slowly, with some grace, finesse and style, like Diane Keaton, Beverly Johnson, Lesley Ann Warren and our great-grandmothers. By that, I mean treat your body right—inside and out—live in great health and support your body as it goes through its normal, natural aging process. Ladies, when you proactively take care of your internal health, your external appearance will truly radiate with that envied youthful glow. I mean it!

"Can I stop crow's-feet in their tracks?"

"Are my mother's age spots normal and am I going to get them?"

"Is it normal to go gray at twenty-seven?"

Good questions.

In this chapter I'm going to show you practical ways to age naturally, gracefully and NOT prematurely. If you are proactive NOW, live the Chill Out and Get Healthy lifestyle and support your body as it goes through its normal aging process, you can have a hot bod, lustrous skin, thick and shiny locks and sturdy nails at the age of fifty.

If you want to stay beautiful, with radiant skin, it's going to take more than that $120 bottle of Peter Thomas Roth's Un-wrinkle. So skip that next cup of coffee, put out that cigarette, ix-nay that Snickers bar, get a decent night's sleep and for crying out loud get on the Chill Out and Get Healthy antiaging train!

Ladies, pick up your currently wattle-free neck and read this next sentence out loud:

**The way my skin looks depends upon
how I treat my body—inside and out.**

In CM we say that beauty has three components: inner, outer and lasting. Or as I have conveniently coined them: **A.C.E.**

- Aesthetic beauty
- Confidence
- Everlasting Beauty

Girl, only when you work on all three A.C.E. components can you truly ace beauty. True beauty is more than just aesthetics; it is a balanced state of radiant health that creates the most fulfilled and beautiful—internally and externally—woman EVER!

Let's break down these three beauty components.

· AESTHETIC BEAUTY ·

Aesthetic beauty is what the outside world sees and is usually what we're most overly OMG-do-I-have-bags-under-my-eyes or can-you-see-my-grays concerned about: our skin, hair and nails. Here's what most people don't get: the appearance of your hair, skin and nails depends upon the efficiency of your body's physiological processes. Your aesthetic beauty depends more on the strength of your digestion and metabolism, the quality of your sleep, how often you poop, the foods you eat and the cleanliness of your liver than on scrubs, cleansers and antiwrinkle creams that cost you your paycheck and fill up your bathroom vanity.

Here are some ancient and priceless recommendations you need to start applying TODAY to make your skin glow, your hair shine and your nails grow strong for years to come.

FAB FOODS

First off, we are going to run through some more general dietary recommendations you all need to follow for internal and external beautification.

"OMG, Aimee! More dietary recommendations!?" I hear you moan.

Listen up: without adequate nourishment, the collagen layers in your aging skin will thin and a degrading, wasting process will take place, leaving you with aged, wrinkled and oh-so-saggy skin. Ladies, without adequate nourishment, your skin will eventually shrivel up like that plant on your windowsill you keep forgetting to water and your hair will fall out, your nails will split and your skin will look like sandpaper. The dietary recs in this chapter are beautifying, nourishing, antiaging and collagen building ... and I know you love that!

Here's how to keep your skin plump and glowing, your hair lush and your nails sturdy:

- **GO ORGANIC.** I know I've said this, like, a gazillion times already, but going organic is imperative. Eat fresh, whole, non-dead, organic foods that are freshly prepared. Yes, organic is more expensive, but just think of how much money you'll save when your skin starts to glow from the inside out and you don't need to buy that hundred-dollar eye cream at Sephora. Apply everything I say in chapters 5 and 6. Do it for your longing-to-be-nourished skin! Just to pound it into your head again: avoid packaged, canned (except for canned light tuna), frozen, processed foods. These foods offer zero nutritional value and do zilch for your aging skin's collagen layers. Not to mention that they are indigestible and create a buildup of toxins inside your body, creating pimples and other gross impurities that show up on your precious skin!

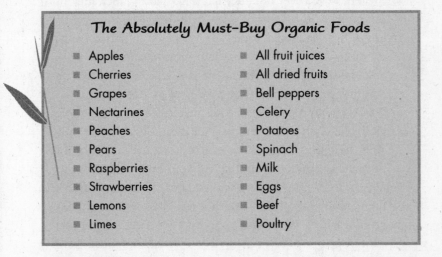

The Absolutely Must-Buy Organic Foods

- Apples
- Cherries
- Grapes
- Nectarines
- Peaches
- Pears
- Raspberries
- Strawberries
- Lemons
- Limes
- All fruit juices
- All dried fruits
- Bell peppers
- Celery
- Potatoes
- Spinach
- Milk
- Eggs
- Beef
- Poultry

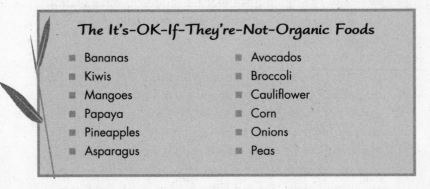

The It's-OK-If-They're-Not-Organic Foods

- Bananas
- Kiwis
- Mangoes
- Papaya
- Pineapples
- Asparagus
- Avocados
- Broccoli
- Cauliflower
- Corn
- Onions
- Peas

- **GO GREEN.** Leafy green vegetables like beet greens (the top part of beets), kale, any kind of seaweed, broccoli, Brussels sprouts, collard greens and spinach nourish the skin and protect it from premature aging. They are loaded with antioxidants (remember, those are the guys that fight off the free radicals that cause aging) and contain many essential vitamins and minerals like iron and calcium that your beautiful body needs daily. And as I said in chapter 7, they also help regulate your hormones! Yummy!
- **SWEETEN UP.** Sweet and juicy fruits like table grapes, melons (all types), pears, plums, grapefruit, oranges, pineapples, kiwis, figs, dates and apples are very rich in antioxidants, promote efficient digestion, help remove impurities from your body and are excellent for the skin. Not to mention that they're great at satisfying your sweet tooth.
- **GRAIN-O-LICIOUS.** Eat a wide variety of organic whole grains, like amaranth, quinoa, millet and barley. Not only are these grains loaded with antioxidants; they are great for promoting healthy poops that rid your body of gross pimple- and cellulite-causing toxins. Did you notice I didn't mention wheat in this list? It's not that organic, stone-ground whole wheat isn't good for you—it is. It's just that a lot of people have a sensitivity to wheat, and wheat isn't as rich in age-fighting antioxidants as other whole grains. Go back and read what I wrote about wheat and gluten sensitivities in chapter 7.
- **LUBE UP.** Use oil and eat butter. Seriously! These types of fats, taken internally, are amazing for the skin. The best oils for you and your skin are organic extra-virgin olive oil, coconut oil (raw, organic and preferably centrifuged) and raw and organic sesame oil. Butters and ghees (clarified butter) that are organic and all-natural should also be included in your diet in moderation, as they lubricate, nourish and create lustrous skin, hair and nails. A word about fat: I know

you are all concerned that eating too much fat will make you fat. Not! Good healthy fats, like the monounsaturated fats found in olive oil, sesame oil and even the saturated fats found in organic butter, are actually great for our health, our skin and our heart! Remember what I said in chapter 6: Fat is good for us! Eat it!

- **SPICE IT UP.** Spices like turmeric, cumin, coriander and red and black pepper can be added to one of your meals or your drinks each day for better health. These yummy spices improve digestion, nourish the skin, detox your liver and cleanse your skin of impurities. Use a half teaspoon, just enough to season your meal or drink, not overpower it. Ingesting too much of these spices in one sitting can upset your tummy, so start small and see how you feel. Turmeric is one of the best antiaging spices for overall health; buy some turmeric tea and drink it a couple of times each week.

- **NO NUKES.** Avoid microwaving and boiling your vegetables. They lose as much as eighty-five percent of their antioxidant content when cooked in this way. If there's more color in the water than there is on the veggie, you've lost the vitamins you so desperately need. Steaming and sautéing are best, but be sure those veggies keep their color.

- **GO NUTS.** Nuts in general are high in the antiaging antioxidant vitamin E and eating them makes one healthy inside and out! Almonds in particular contain high concentrations of antioxidants, ward off sugar cravings and help reduce cholesterol. Brazil nuts are extremely rich in selenium, an antioxidant linked to lower rates of heart disease and cancer. Walnuts contain ellagic acid, an antioxidant and a cancer fighter, and are also high in omega-3-type oil. If you are allergic to nuts, plan on getting your omega-3 and antioxidants from foods like olive oil, avocados and organic eggs.

TOP TEN, ABSOLUTE-BEST-EVER, ANTIOXIDANT-RICH, SKIN-BEAUTIFYING FOODS

OK, now let's get even more specific. Hands down, the following are my top ten absolute-best-ever, antioxidant-rich, skin-beautifying, must-eat-daily foods. They're nature's antiaging rock stars that battle wrinkles, pimples, sun damage, cellulite and wattly neck horrors! Eat these foods regularly, organic when possible. I recommend getting in at least one of these foods each day of the week (and you can eat a small handful of nuts or flaxseeds EVERY day of the week). Mix it up, rotate them, follow my serving-size advice and don't overdo it. Remember, too much of a good thing isn't always good.

1. **AVOCADOS.** An avocado a day keeps the premature aging demons away. This luscious fruit (yes, it's a fruit) is the highest in the antiwrinkle, antipimple, anticellulite, vitamin E department. If that weren't enough, the avocado is also a prime source of the antioxidant glutathione, an antioxidant that's responsible for deterring the development of skin cancer. Eat three to four avocados a week (remember, they don't need to be organic); put them in your salads, your protein shakes or some homemade guac (see my recipe in chapter 6!). You can even put overripe avocados on your hair for a nourishing hair mask. Don't worry about the fat; it's good for you and it's amazing for your skin (and hair).

2. **GREEN TEA.** Green tea is skin's best friend. It's loaded with polyphenols that protect your skin from inflammation associated with exposure to ultraviolet light, and helps prevent skin cancer! Have a cup of organic green tea every day. Good brands to buy are Tazo and Yogi. Or go to a local tea shop and buy organic green tea in bulk.

3. **SWEET POTATOES.** Sweet potatoes are an all-around antiaging nutritional goddess. They are packed with vitamins C and E and are one of nature's greatest sources of beta-carotene. According to a study published in the *European Jour-*

nal of *Dermatology*, beta-carotene's ability to absorb light may protect skin by minimizing sunburn. Once digested, beta-carotene converts to vitamin A, a nutrient that plays a major role in promoting healthy skin. Vitamin A is critical to maintaining skin integrity in addition to warding off wrinkle-causing oxidative stress. Without it, skin becomes rough, dry and scaly. Eat an organic sweet potato at least once per week, roasted, baked, sautéed or pureed in a soup. And while you're at it, add a dab of organic butter or ghee.

4. **BLUEBERRIES.** Blueberries are bite-sized antioxidant and anticancer machines. To boot, they're high in vitamin C, which is instrumental for the synthesis of collagen, one of the skin's major structural wrinkle-fighting proteins. We love ANYTHING that promotes natural collagen synthesis! When they're in season, eat a cup of fresh blueberries daily. When they aren't in season, buy frozen blueberries (preferably organic) and make a smoothie.

5. **GOJI BERRIES.** These little guys have been a part of CM's herbal regimen for thousands of years! They are the über-antioxidant with five hundred times more vitamin C per ounce than oranges. Goji berries also contain linoleic acid, an essential fatty acid that plumps up the skin and makes it look smooth, supple and youthful. Go goji. A handful of goji berries (preferably organic) each day is plenty. No need to overdo it.

6. **FLAXSEEDS.** This seed is packed with omega-3 fatty acids, which are crucial to amazing skin. One of the omega-3 fatty acids it contains is alpha-linolenic acid (ALA), which helps keep skin smooth and pliable. Flaxseed is the best source of plant omega-3 fats (although fish, specifically fish oil, is the best overall source of omega-3). Remember what I said in chapter 7: be sure to eat the seeds and not the oil. Sprinkle them on your favorite foods like your organic steel-cut oatmeal, your full-fat organic yogurt or your fruit smoothies. You can eat a tablespoon or two of flaxseeds daily.

7. **TOMATOES.** Not only are tomatoes rich in collagen-building vitamin C; they also contain the major antioxidant lycopene. FYI: lycopene is also found in watermelon and Ruby Red grapefruit. Eat as many tomatoes (preferably organic) as you want. Slice and sprinkle with organic sea salt and olive oil for an afternoon snack.

8. **WALNUTS.** When it comes to fat, there are two kinds we need that our body can't make—linoleic and linolenic acids. Leave these out of your diet, and your skin will be dry and flaky—eeewww! While most of us eat plenty of linoleic acid (found in veggies, fruits [including goji berries], nuts, grains and seeds), it is a lot harder to get enough linolenic acid (found in flaxseeds, walnuts, pumpkin seeds, spirulina and green leafy veggies). That's where walnuts come in. They are packed with beta-carotene and vitamin E and alpha-linolenic acid, helping to keep skin soft, smooth and supple. Walnuts also contain zinc, which plays a pivotal role in healing aged and injured or acne-ridden skin. Eat a handful of organic walnuts a day.

9. **MEDICINAL MUSHROOMS.** Eat medicinal mushrooms, namely, maitake, shiitake, reishi (aka ganoderm lucidum or ling zhi) and wood ear (aka black mushrooms). These mushrooms are kick-ass antiaging, skin-rejuvenating, essence-generating foods that have been a part of CM healing tradition for centuries. Put them in your salads, sauté them with some sesame oil or drizzle some olive oil on them and munch on them raw. Just eat 'em!

10. **OLIVE OIL.** I remember being in Greece one summer, talking with my best girlfriend's eighty-year-old grandmother, who had the most amazingly supple and smooth skin. When I said, "You have such beautiful skin," she smiled and said, "Olive oil." That's it? Since the age of fourteen she's been putting only olive oil on her skin each morning and night (and of course she's been ingesting it for longer than that). In 2001,

Australian researchers concluded that individuals who consumed diets rich in olive oil had the most youthful-looking skin. Why? It seems that olive oil's high monounsaturated-fat content keeps skin cells in tip-top shape by preventing injury to the outer shell of skin cells. Couple that with generous proportions of vitamin E, polyphenols and beta-carotene, and you've got an antiaging powerhouse! So put it in your salads and then dab some on a cotton ball and put it on your clean face before you go to bed at night. Use it daily (if it suits your skin type—we'll discuss that in detail later on in this chapter). Buy it organic. And before you cook with it, go over what I said in chapter 6 about cooking with olive oil.

FAB FEMALE SKIN TYPES

Besides dietary recommendations, another major key to aesthetic beauty is understanding your skin type according to CM principles. Chinese Medicine recognizes three different skin types: Earth, Wind and Fire. Yes, just like the popular seventies R & B group.

So let's figure out which type you are. Read about each of the types, Earth Girls, Windy City Girls and Fire Girls; then decide which one you are, follow the recommendations I make for your type and then rock out with your new-you fabulous skin!

EARTH GIRLS

Famous Earth Girls:
Norah Jones, Catherine Zeta-Jones and Renée Zellweger

Earth types have thick, oily and soft skin that is cool to the touch. Their faces are full and moonlike, and their hair is thick, wavy, oily and often dark in color.

Earth Girl types are lucky bitches. Innately they have more collagen and connective tissue than the rest of us and they usually don't develop wrinkles until much later in life.

The woes of Earth's skin

When Earth Girl's skin is out of balance, she will have enlarged pores, excessively oily skin, moist types of eczema (the kind that seeps a clear fluid), blackheads, pimples, cellulite and water retention. Imbalanced Earth Girls are also more prone to fungal infections and sagging jowls.

Getting Earth Girl's skin back on track

- Avoid greasy, clogging creams because your pores love to clog up. Go for organic, paraben-free, chemical-free, water-based foundations, like those found at suncoatproducts.com, yvesrocherusa.com and econveybeauty.com. (You'll find more information on going green with your skin care and makeup at the end of this chapter.)
- Clean your face regularly with plain old water and a clean facecloth. If you can, rinse your face in the morning, afternoon and evening, even if that means reapplying (all-natural, chemical-free) makeup during the day.
- Avoid heavy, hard-to-digest foods like fried foods, fatty meats, cheeses and rich dairy-based desserts. Besides the fact that for the most part these foods are ridiculously unhealthy for you, they'll give the Earth Girl type pimples and cellulite (which they're already more prone to). Don't eat them!
- Limit your dairy (milk, yogurt and cheese) intake. Keep it down to three very small three-ounce servings a week. Instead get your calcium from green, leafy veggies. If you recall from chapter 5, one cup of cooked spinach, turnips or collard greens gives you just as much calcium as one cup of milk. Sesame seeds are also a great source of calcium for you; sprinkle them on your salad, yogurt (when you have one) or oatmeal and put some in your smoothies.
- Avoid overly sweet fruits like mangoes, pineapples, grapes, bananas and dates, as their overwhelming, albeit natural, sweetness can hamper your digestion and cause you to re-

tain more water. Plain and simple, even these natural foods are just too sweet for the Earth Girl.

- Avoid salt, another thing that will cause you to retain more water than non–Earth Girl types.
- Astringent, bitter and pungent foods like bok choy, bell peppers, daikon radish, eggplant, onion, ginger, mustard seed and citrus fruits should be your best friend, as they balance your skin tremendously and keep it from getting clogged up and pimply. These types of foods assist your naturally slow digestion and thereby prevent toxins from building up in your system.
- Avoid cold or frozen foods or smoothies, as they will slow down your digestion and metabolism even more. Sure, in the hot summer months a smoothie once or twice a week is fine, but in the colder months Earth Girls should steer clear of cold or frozen foods (remember how I said in chapter 2 how cold foods will slow down digestion?). Instead, put fresh fruit and room-temperature water in your smoothies; they'll taste just as good and won't (literally) freeze up your metabolism.
- Have nuts in moderation, as they are a bit too fatty and oily for your skin type. Instead get your omega-3 from flaxseeds, sesame seeds, olive oil, fish and organic eggs.
- Have a mug of hot water with a little slice of fresh ginger and some fresh lime juice before meals. The astringent quality of lime is great for your skin, and the warm nature of ginger will increase your characteristically slow metabolism.
- Drink fifty ounces of room-temperature water per day. Unlike women with the other skin types, you are prone to water retention and bloating, so you shouldn't have as much water as Fire and Wind Girls. Obviously on a hot day, or if you're really thirsty, it's OK to drink more. Just know that your body has a tendency toward water retention.
- Take warm baths often, using Epsom salts. The salts will help keep your body from retaining excess water.

- Use gentle skin cleansers, like Cetaphil, Weleda's wild rose cleansing lotion or Burt's Bees orange essence facial cleanser to open and purify your pores.
- Make it your business to poop daily; otherwise the toxins in your colon will creep up and make your skin oily and puffy.
- Get some exercise every day to increase circulation and help purify the skin through the sweating process.

Earth Girl's very own facial oil

Weleda's wild rose facial oil (you can purchase this at most health-food stores, or USA.Weleda.com). Important: test the oil on a small patch of skin, up near your scalp, to be sure your skin doesn't react negatively to it.

Why I LOVE Weleda

Since 1921, Weleda has been a pioneer in the facial-care industry, using only organic ingredients. They support local farmers and sustainable organic agriculture. They NEVER use chemicals and their products ROCK!
www.usa.weleda.com

Earth Girl's face mask

Ingredients
1 organic egg white (if you are allergic to eggs, substitute raw—not toasted—sesame or olive oil)
½ fresh lemon
1 vial of pearl powder
2 drops of cypress essential oil (be sure to test this oil on your skin to make certain your skin doesn't react negatively to it before you apply the mask)

Directions
Separate the egg, and put the white in a small bowl . Take

your ½ lemon and squeeze all the juice out of it into your bowl. Then add your vial of pearl powder and the cypress oil. Mix with a spoon. After all ingredients are mixed thoroughly, take a cotton ball and apply the mask to your freshly cleaned face, avoiding your eyes and any open sores, pimples or newly waxed upper lip/eyebrow areas (the lemon will sting!). Lie down, chill out and let your mask dry (about 10 minutes). Wash your face with warm water. Dry your face and apply a thin layer of your fragrant and astringent wild rose facial oil.

What this mask will do for the Earth Girl

Both the lemon and the cypress oil are astringent and very good for removing impurities and excess fluids from your skin. The pearl powder is an all-around beauty powerhouse and will make your skin shine like a radiant pearl.

Precious Pearl Powder

Legend has it that a Chinese empress renowned for her youthful skin crushed a pearl and used a stick of jade to rub it on her wrinkles—smoothing them away. Pearl powder contains amino acids and trace elements that rejuvenate your skin. You can find it at Chinese herb stores; look for the Chinese name *zhen zhu*, or the pharmaceutical name Margarita. You can purchase pearl powder online at radiantpearlskin.com.

WINDY CITY GIRLS

Famous Windy City Girls:
Sarah Jessica Parker, Jennifer Aniston and Beyoncé Knowles

The Wind skin type has dry, thin, fine-pored and sensitive skin that is cool to the touch. When balanced, the Wind Girl's skin glows with a delicate lightness that is elegant and attractive. When Wind skin is out of whack, it is prone to excessive dryness and may even be rough and flaky, including the scalp.

The woes of Wind's skin

The greatest woe facing the Windy City Girl is a predisposition to symptoms of early aging. Ahhh!! Your skin may develop wrinkles earlier than most, due to its tendency toward dryness and thinness. Since your skin does not contain much moisture, preventing it from drying is your major job. If your digestion is not in balance, your skin can begin to look dull and grayish, even in your twenties and thirties.

In addition, your skin may have a tendency toward dry eczema and skin fungus. Excess worry and fear will also show on your face. And if you're not sleeping seven-plus hours each night, your skin will look tired and lifeless. Windy City G: eat clean, keep your skin nourished and poop daily.

Getting Windy City Girl's skin back on track

- Eat lots of healthy fats and oils (like avocados, salmon, coconut milk, coconut oil and olive oil). Have two servings of a healthy fat or oil a day. Cook with olive or coconut oil, put some olive oil or avocado on a salad, eat some salmon. . . . You get it, right?
- Eat full-fat yogurt and milk. Have five four-ounce servings per week (but not all in the form of milk—try for three servings of yogurt/week and one of milk), because the fat and the dairy are good for you and nourishing to your body, inside and out.
- Eat sour foods like lemons, grapefruit or pomegranates daily, because they are very detoxifying and will help you poop.
- Start off each day with a mug of hot water with half a fresh-squeezed lemon and a teaspoon of all-natural raw honey. It's überdetoxifying for you.
- Use a dash or two of salt a day on your food. Or eat a pickle a day. Salt, in moderation, is good, as it retains water and nourishes skin that is prone to drying.

- Have two servings of sweet fruit per day (like goji berries, blueberries, plums, bananas or dates). The sweet flavor balances the dryness associated with the Wind element. Do not substitute with unnatural sugars (yellow, blue or pink packets are bad!), as these substances are inflammatory and will make your skin dry, red and itchy.
- Avoid drying, wheat-based foods like crackers, pastas, processed white or whole wheat breads or pretzels.
- Drink half your body weight in ounces of room-temperature water per day (for example, if you weigh 130 pounds, you should be drinking 65 ounces of water). Water that is colder than room temperature is too cold for your body type and may upset your stomach and slow down your digestion.
- Get your butt to bed early—before ten p.m.—and sleep! Sleep is very soothing for your skin type and it will show. This is important for all skin types, but imperative for yours. If you can't get to bed by ten, just be sure you are getting seven to eight hours of uninterrupted sleep each night.
- Avoid cleansing products that dry the skin (like alcohol-based cleansers or toners). Clean with nourishing cleansers like organic olive oil soap, Cetaphil or Weleda's iris cleansing lotion.
- Massage either organic olive oil or coconut oil onto your whole body in the morning after you shower. This is oh-so-nourishing. If your scalp is particularly dry, apply my Ahh-vo Nourishing Hair Mask once a week. Let it soak into your scalp for a half hour and then wash out. I swear it won't make your hair a greasy wild wreck. The oils and fats will wash right out with one rinse and it will leave your hair and scalp supple-icious.

. . .

Ahh-vo Nourishing Hair Mask

1 egg yolk
2 tablespoons olive oil
2 tablespoons mayonnaise
1 avocado

Mix all ingredients together in a bowl and apply to your scalp and hair, particularly the ends. Put on a shower cap and chill for a half hour. Then rinse your hair.

Windy City Girl's facial oil

Raw, organic and centrifuged coconut oil (you can buy this online at wildernessfamilynaturals.com or greenpasture.org, or in most health-food stores), organic olive oil or organic apricot-kernel oil (Aura Cacia makes a great one).

Windy City Girl's face mask

Ingredients

¼ cup brown sugar
2 drops of organic lavender essential oil (test this oil on your skin to make sure your skin doesn't react negatively to it before you apply the mask)
2 tablespoons organic goat's milk
1 vial of pearl powder

Directions

In a small bowl mix all your ingredients thoroughly. Using your clean fingers and a clean cotton ball, apply mixture to your freshly cleaned face. Lie down, chill out and leave the mask on for 10 minutes. This mask won't dry. Rinse your face with warm water. Apply a thin layer of apricot-kernel oil to your towel-dried face.

• • •

What this mask will do for the Windy City Girl

This mask will nourish your skin and ward off its tendency toward premature aging, dryness and irritation. The fat from the goat's milk is loaded with nourishment for your skin; the lavender is soothing and calming for your skin; the brown sugar is nourishing and enriching for your skin type and will help ward off the signs of premature aging; the pearl powder is a beauty powerhouse and will make your skin shine and glow.

> Goat's milk has been used as a skin rejuvenator for centuries. It's loaded with proteins, calcium and fatty acids. In fact, Cleopatra used to bathe in goat's milk to maintain her radiant skin.
>
> With the leftover goat's milk, you can be like Cleopatra and bathe in it, you can put it on your scalp for a nourishing treatment or you can drink it. It's great inside and outside.

FIRE GIRLS

Famous Fire Girls:
Lindsay Lohan, Lucy Liu and Shakira

The Fire Girl has fair, soft and warm skin that is on the thicker side. When her skin is happy, it has a beautiful glow and her cheeks are rosy. Her hair is typically fine and straight, and is usually red, sandy or blond in color. Fire Girls tend to have a pink or reddish complexion and a good amount of freckles or moles.

The woes of Fire's skin

Fire types tend to develop rashes, rosacea, acne, liver spots and/or pigment disorders. Of the three skin types, Fire Girl has the least tolerance for the sun and will show signs of sun damage as she ages. As well, Fire skin is aggravated by emotional stress, especially suppressed anger, frustration or resentment. If you're a Fire

Girl, it's insanely important for you to express your emotions—your skin is at stake!

Getting Fire Girl's skin back on track

- Avoid excessive sunlight, tanning treatments and highly heating therapies like facial or whole-body steams.
- Avoid hot, spicy foods and seasonings like chilies and cayenne peppers, as these are fiery foods and will aggravate your skin (and your repressed anger!). Opt for spices such as turmeric, coriander, cinnamon and fennel.
- Drink organic green tea daily with half a fresh-squeezed lemon in it, as this will help move your bowels and keep your Fire side at bay. You can get decaffeinated green tea.
- Eat astringent and sour foods like lemons, grapefruit, limes, pears, plums, tangerines or pomegranates twice daily. They are very detoxifying and will help you poop.
- Eat lots of bitter green leafy veggies like spinach, broccoli rabe, beet greens, dandelion greens, sprouts and cabbage, because they are very cleansing and cooling to your overheated and easily irritated bod. They're also great for PMS!
- Eat four servings of naturally sweet foods like grapes, coconuts, cherries, melons, mangoes, plums and pineapples a week. The sweet flavor balances Fire, but you don't want to overdo it, as too much sweetness can aggravate the Fire-type skin.
- Do not eat refined sugary sweet foods, as they are very inflammatory and will aggravate your skin and make it red and blotchy.
- Drinking plenty of water helps wash impurities from sensitive Fire skin. Because of your Fire side, having cool or cold water is OK for you. Divide your body weight in half and drink that many ounces of water per day.
- Use a sensitive and delicate face cleanser like Weleda's almond cleansing lotion.
- Keep your emotional stress under control through plenty of outdoor exercise, yoga and meditation.

Fire Girl's facial oil

Raw (not toasted) organic sesame oil (Aura Cacia makes a good one) or Weleda's almond facial oil.

Fire Girl's face mask

Ingredients
¼ cup organic green tea

1 organic egg white (if you are allergic to eggs, substitute raw—not toasted—sesame or olive oil)

1 tablespoon turmeric powder

1 vial of pearl powder

Directions
Heat up your teakettle and add ¼ cup of boiling water to 1 organic green tea bag. Steep for 2 minutes. Toss the tea bag. Let the green tea cool down. In a small bowl, mix the egg white with the COOLED green tea (otherwise the egg will cook). Add the turmeric and pearl powder. Mix thoroughly. Apply mixture to your freshly cleaned face with a cotton ball. Lie down, chill out and let the mask dry (about 10 minutes). Wash your face with warm water. Apply a thin layer of sesame oil to your freshly cleaned towel-dried face.

What this mask will do for the Fire Girl
This mask will both cool the "fire" in your skin (i.e., redness, rosacea and rashes) and improve the circulation in your skin, thereby balancing your complexion. The turmeric is great for promoting circulation and the green tea is very cooling. The pearl powder will make your skin shine and radiate. You'll love how balanced your skin looks after you apply this mask.

. . .

> ### The Healing Powers of Turmeric
>
> Turmeric has been used for centuries in Chinese Medicine. It has natural anti-inflammatory, anticancer, liver-detoxifying, wound-healing and incredible circulatory properties. You can buy it in powder form from itoen.com; most health-food stores should carry it too.

• CONFIDENCE •

Now that we've thoroughly covered the aesthetics of A.C.E.-ing your beauty, let's move on to an essential element of beauty: confidence.

"Confidence, schmonfidence, Aimee! Give me more ancient beauty secrets!"

Ladies, hear me out. Happy, positive, loving and confident people have a glowing beauty that is far more than skin-deep. You can see it yourself. On a day when you're on a high over a new job promotion, a hot new date or a new pair of sexy jeans, you are beaming, your skin looks fabulous and strangers give you compliments. On the other end of the spectrum, when you're feeling stressed-out, tired and ho-hum, what types of comments do people proffer? They say things like "You look tired," "You need some sun," "You should get yourself a massage" or, the best one yet, "Girl, you need to get laid!"

Get it? Onlookers sure do.

For thousands of years, it has been known that confidence creates beauty. The authentic quality of confidence is the oldest beauty secret in the book. No bronzer or shimmery blush can create it. Not even highlights, lowlights or a blowout can produce that internal shine that comes from a truly confident woman. A woman who is genuinely confident and owns her I-am-woman-hear-me-roar goods from the inside out has a glow that cannot be found in any beauty product or magazine article.

Woman, you need confidence with where you are in your life, careerwise, relationshipwise, bodywise, healthwise. If you don't love and accept yourself right here, right now, it doesn't matter what beauty tip you apply; you will always be missing something. Be vigilant, take control of your life, make the changes you want to make and find your inner confidence. Roar like the mighty woman you are and glow from the inside out!

"How, Aimee?" I hear you moan. "I thought I was glowing already!"

Now, that's an ancient secret you deserve to know. In CM theory, confidence comes from a mind and heart that are in harmony. A woman with her mind and heart in harmony speaks her truth, expresses—not represses—her emotions, manages her stress, goes for what she wants and has the ability to find peace every day. Confidence comes from a woman who knows how to CTFO and does it on a daily basis. Confidence comes from a woman who sets her sights on her goal and just dives in.

Keys to maintaining your confidence are found throughout this book, particularly in chapter 4, the best tool being the "Mirror, Mirror" exercise. For a confidence booster, we can put a spin on the self-talk exercise: each night when you are in your bathroom washing your face, I want you to look in the mirror and find one thing you don't like about your appearance. Maybe it's your eyebrow furrow, your nose or a newfound blemish. Maybe it's your body shape, your thighs, your hips, your belly or your boobs. Maybe it's something one can't see, like your boyfriend or your unfulfilling job. Find just one thing. Then say to yourself in the mirror, in a loving, compassionate and accepting way:

"I love and accept _____ [fill in the blank with your issue], this part of myself. This _____ [insert issue here] is part of who I am and I love ALL of me. I accept myself as I am now. I am a confident and beautiful woman. I am woman, hear me ROAR!"

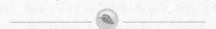

Samantha, a thirty-three-year-old TV producer, came to me for help with her "adult acne." She wanted help ASAP, as this acne was killing her ego.

She was an obvious Earth Girl, with large pores, oily skin and NO wrinkles! She struggled with constipation and had an easy time gaining weight. Her period was regular—she had no complaints about it—her energy levels were good, she exercised regularly and she was getting eight hours of restful sleep each night.

Her diet had way too much dairy in it (she was eating eight or more ounces each day) and practically no green veggies.

For skin care, she was using a harsh, chemical-laden exfoliator several times per day, an oil-free (but paraben-plenty) moisturizer and layers of foundation to cover up her acne.

I had her cut back on dairy, start drinking rice milk, eat more green veggies and drink a mug of hot water with ginger and lime juice each morning. And—wouldn't you know it?—she started going to the bathroom every morning.

I directed her to wash her face with only water and to stop using so much foundation. She used Burt's Bees facial scrub every other day and did the Earth Girl face mask four nights a week.

She started saying "I love you" to herself in the mirror, every single day. It took a month or so, but her skin cleared up and she had a confident internal glow.

Keep doing this on a regular basis until there are no more "issues" to find.

And always remember to look into the mirror, deep into your own eyes, and say, "I love you!"

Call me crazy, but it will work. Look deep into your own eyes and let yourself know that no matter what wrinkle or blemish or bad job, you will always love and accept yourself. You will always be beautiful and confident. Even if you don't believe it at this moment, talk yourself into it. You can do it.

All women, even the Giseles and the Jen Anistons, have something about their internal and external appearance they may not like. It's part of human nature. But if you don't love and accept yourself entirely—blemishes, big butt and all—you'll be missing a key element to your outer beauty: inner confidence. Not to mention that once you own that inner confidence, you will have the gall to make the changes your life is longing for—like treating your insides right, getting to the gym more often or reinvigorating your career.

Girl, it's time you seriously worked on building and sustaining your inner confidence. Give yourself a nightly pep talk. Love and accept yourself. Work on yourself by regularly using the tools in chapter 4. Oh, and don't forget to eat clean, do your face mask, follow the recommendations for your skin type, poop daily, drink lots of water, express yourself and sleep! It sounds like a lot of work, but you can do it. Just pace yourself. One step at a time—you don't have to do it all at once. Just start NOW.

• EVERLASTING BEAUTY •

Now on to the final element of beauty, the one we all dream about: everlasting beauty. Also known as being hot like Madonna at fifty (without the need for a personal trainer, stylist and chef).

In order to understand how to make our beauty everlasting, we must first learn what truly ages us. One ancient CM beauty secret goes like this:

At the age of forty, the mind is visible on the face.

Ladies, what this ancient principle is saying is that the way in which we live our lives will one day, very soon, show up on our face. Oh dear! Said another way, if you're happy and healthy and confident and content, you'll look that way. You'll glow and others will admire your inner and outer beauty. However, if you live with discontent and regret, party like a rock star, get very little sleep and live on Red Bull or Dunkin' Donuts Coffee Coolattas—it will show on your face and in your body. Sooner than you think.

"What do I do, Aimee?"

You're already doing it. By reading this book you have made a choice. You are choosing prevention. You are choosing health NOW. Sure, Botox or Restylane injections or plastic surgery may seem a reasonable way to battle this aging process, for some. But whatever happened to aging au naturel with grace and style? I know that all of us want to look hot and refreshed at fifty. Do we really have to go under the knife or inject noxious substances into our bodies to do so? NO. In order to slow the aging process, remain sexy, glow from the inside out and have the confidence you deserve, you MUST treat your outsides well, treat your insides even better, express your emotions and live with contentment and peace. If you don't, it will show on your face and body and in your lack of health!

I'd be lying if I said the CM way to everlasting beauty doesn't take work. Work is the opposite of making an appointment with your derm to get an injection. However, if you do the work, you will reap the rewards, without needles filled with gross chemicals being stuck in your face. Where do you think the anger or worry that created that wrinkle in your forehead goes after that injection of Botox makes it disappear? And why do you think the wrinkle keeps coming back after the Botox wears off? These wrinkles are present because there are internal factors producing them and those factors need to be resolved; anything else and you are just covering up the symptom, not caring for the root problem. There are issues that you need to look at. All of us have them—me included. There are things in your life that need work. You can do it. Go back to chapter 4 and work on you. Eat clean. Follow my recommendations for your skin type. You deserve it. Your inner self deserves it. Your face deserves it.

Girls, everlasting beauty is an internal and external process. I'm gonna burst your bubble right now: everlasting beauty doesn't come in a five-hundred-dollar botulism shot. And it definitely doesn't come in a ten-thousand-dollar face-lift. What you get is a dependence on these treatments, which are costly, risky and ridiculously far from au naturel.

Here's a five-point summary of what you have to do to acquire everlasting beauty. (I know most of the following have already been discussed ad nauseam in this book, but I told you from the get-go that I was going to pound these recommendations into your head until I'm blue in the face. So here I go, yet again.)

1. Live clean: beauty's ever-last-ability is completely and totally dependent upon how you treat the insides and outsides of your body. That means, don't put chemically processed commercial-pesticide-ridden food into your body and don't put chemically treated synthetic animal-abusing makeup or products on your face, in your hair or on your nails. These toxins undoubtedly contribute to premature aging and will make your skin sag and wrinkle. Period.

2. Sleep! Get your butt to bed by ten p.m. This simple habit is one of the most powerful techniques for health and longevity. If you can't get to sleep by ten, then be sure to at least get seven to eight hours of uninterrupted sleep.

3. CTFO daily. I know I sound like a broken record. Just freakin' do it! Your everlasting beauty will thank you!

4. Follow the recommendations for your skin type and do your facial masks as often as possible. You could even CTFO while you are resting with your mask on. I know you: you're all about multitasking.

5. Be confident. Roar like the woman that you are. Say "I love you" to yourself every day! Work on you. Iron out the kinks. Be content. Find peace in your heart. Of course, this is easier said than done, but just keep at it. Evolving into the confident and beautiful woman you long to be is a process. Don't give up on it, don't give up on you!

Everyone's unique beauty shines forth when they have radiant health and personal happiness. Beauty is a side effect of a balanced, fulfilled and expressive life. Beauty is not a gift. It's a choice! Make it! Be smart, live clean and make the choice to A.C.E. your personal beauty.

Ladies, remember:

Aesthetic Beauty + Confidence = Everlasting Beauty

"Needles in my face? No way!"

Hey, I do it. All my girlfriends do it. You should do it! It works and leaves you feeling and looking amazingly rejuvenated!

How does it work?

Facial-rejuvenation acupuncture uses acupuncture, Chinese herbs and lifestyle modifications to rebalance your facial circulation and soften the signs of aging. It's a painless, nonsurgical process that improves facial muscle tone, revitalizes aging skin and visibly improves your appearance by detoxifying your mind and body. Facial acupuncture works on both an energetic and a physical level—reducing bags and sagging around the eyes, tightening the sagging skin around the neck, plumping the apples of your cheeks, diminishing fine lines and wrinkles and restoring your youthful radiant glow.

Bottom line—it's awesome!

To find a qualified practitioner in your area, check out Aimee Raupp.com.

· MORE ANCIENT AESTHETIC TREATMENT ·
FOR WHAT AILS YOU

The following are great topical treatments for common beauty issues according to CM principles.

- **DARK UNDER-EYE CIRCLES.** Mix one tablespoon of turmeric powder with one tablespoon of honey. Apply the goop under your eyes. Leave on for ten minutes. Turmeric is a very powerful blood circulator and will invigorate your under-eye complexion, diminishing dark circles. Before you apply the tumeric mixture under your eyes, apply a small amount to an area of skin near your scalp, or on your neck—leave it for a few minutes just to be sure you don't have an allergic reaction to turmeric.

- **ACNE.** Make a lemon and egg-white mask. Whisk one egg white with the juice from a fresh lemon. Apply to your face. Leave on for ten minutes, then rinse off with warm water. Lemon is a very astringent fruit with natural antibiotic activity. It will help to topically reduce acne.
- **GENERAL BEAUTIFICATION FOR A HOT DATE.** This mask is a no-brainer for any girl wanting a quick glow. Mix one vial of pearl powder with two tablespoons of olive oil, sesame oil, almond oil or apricot-kernel oil. Mix and apply a thin layer to your face. Let it soak for ten minutes. Rinse with warm water.
- **THINNING HAIR.** Juice up some gingerroot and mix it with white wine vinegar (a fifty-fifty ratio). Take a cotton ball and apply to your hair nightly. Keep this potion in the fridge. Ginger and vinegar are both very invigorating and help hair regrowth. I've used this extensively with patients, and it really works!! Another great tool for helping hair grow thick and luscious is brushing your hair for twenty minutes a day with a natural-bristle hairbrush (Kent makes some great natural-bristle hairbrushes). You can do this while you are sitting in front of the TV or just hanging out at home. The natural bristles both stimulate hair-growing blood flow to your scalp and pull your hair's oil through the hair shaft, making it strong and shiny. Give it a shot.
- **NAIL FUNGUS.** Take four drops of oregano oil (you can find this at most health-food stores) and mix it in four ounces of any other oil (olive and sesame are great choices). Stir it up and apply to the affected area. Be sure to mix the oregano oil with a carrier oil, as it will burn your skin if it's not diluted.
- **ECZEMA.** Being an eczema sufferer myself, I know how aggravating this skin issue can be.
    - ◆ Weepy, wet eczema: either buy powdered oats (Aveeno makes some) or take some oatmeal and grind it to powder in a coffee-bean grinder. Mix one table-

spoon of oatmeal powder with one egg white and a couple of drops of lavender. Apply it to the area and let it dry for about ten minutes. Rinse and reapply as needed. It's very soothing.

- Dry eczema: apply coconut oil to it as often as possible. Weleda also makes a great lotion called Skin Food that works beautifully on dry eczema.

- **CELLULITE**
  - Drink barley water with lemon.

    "What's barley water?" you ask.

    Girl, you're going to make yourself some. Go out and buy a bag of pearled barley. Simmer one-half cup of the pearled barley in one quart of water for twenty minutes. If the barley water becomes too thick to drink comfortably, add more water. Remove from the stove and sieve off the water (the grain can be saved for a soup or a salad). Add the juice from two lemons to your homemade barley water. Drink one to two cups per day. Barley water is very cleansing to the body and particularly works on removing the extracellular debris in your body that causes cellulite.

  - Get yourself a body brush. This is great for assisting the body in ridding itself of toxic cellular debris that causes cellulite. Always brush toward your heart, as this is the way the lymph system flows and the lymph nodes are the guys that get clogged and render you cellulite-ish.

- **DRY AND LIFELESS HAIR.** Do the Ahh-vo Nourishing Hair Mask. Mix one egg yolk, two tablespoons of olive oil, two tablespoons of mayonnaise and one avocado in a bowl and apply to your scalp and hair, particularly the ends. Put on a shower cap and chill for a half hour. Then rinse your hair. It's ahh-mazing!

- **DRY AND DANDRUFFY SCALP.** Soak your scalp with olive oil or coconut oil. Leave on overnight (you may want to wear a nightcap to bed so as not to damage your sheets). Rinse the oil off in the morning. Shampoo as usual.

- **FOR OVERALL LUSCIOUS SKIN.** Bathe in organic goat's milk, just like Cleopatra. If a whole bathtub filled with goat's milk is a bit excessive, just take some goat's milk, and using a cotton cloth, apply to your body after a hot shower. Then rinse. Yummy.

· THE LOWDOWN ON MAKEUP · AND BEAUTY PRODUCTS

A lot of companies that make your beauty products (including Estée Lauder, Avon, OPI, L'Oréal, Revlon, Procter & Gamble and Unilever) use toxic chemicals like lead, formaldehyde and lanolin that are B-A-D for your skin (see box on pages 203–4)! Even though you are not ingesting these products (I hope!), you are still absorbing the chemically toxic nonsense through the largest organ in your body: your skin. There are a lot of evil beauty products out there. Be an educated consumer. Use the list in the box "The Most Common Toxic Chemicals in Your Skin-Care Products" and check out the products in your vanity. Toss any product that contains any of the scary chemicals listed! Yes, it may be a waste of hard-earned money, but your health and your skin are worth it! Right?

I know that going green with your makeup and skin care may seem like a bit much. But if you're going to go green on the inside, then you should really go green with your outsides too. With companies like Weleda and Burt's Bees, it's not that hard to make the switch with your skin care. The hardest part, and I know this personally, is to give up the makeup lines we've been attached to for the last ten years. So, girls, what do we do?

Well, this is what I did.

First, I started with my skin-care lines. I switched completely over to Weleda, Aura Cacia and Avalon Organics products. You can too. Just follow the recommendations I give for your skin type in this chapter. Get rid of all the harsh cleansers, toners and exfoliators that you own.

I switched to Aubrey and Burt's Bees products for my shampoo and conditioner.

Next, I went to the Environmental Working Group's Skin Deep: Cosmetic Safety Database (www.cosmeticsdatabase.com) and searched for the makeup I was using before I decided to go green. This database ranks makeup products on a scale of one to ten on their safety (one being the safest). Using their easy search engine, I found that some of my favorite products contained cancer-causing and reproductively toxic agents. Yuck! So I browsed their makeup section (which lists products, product types and safety level) and found products that were safe and similar to the ones I was using. My rule of thumb was to not go above a two on the safety level. I switched from Benefit's liquid foundation to Tarte's; I switched my mascara, concealer, bronzer and lip gloss to safer versions. Browsing the hair-care section of the database, I even found that Bumble and Bumble makes a great nontoxic styling gel that works better than the toxic one I was using. Girl, get on the Web site and search for your products. It wasn't hard and it'll make you feel and look fabulous with a truly healthy and environmentally safe glow!

The basic truth is that chemicals aren't good for our skin, hair and nails and they are definitely not good for our environment. Not to get all "power to the people" on you, but if we made a stand and stopped supporting these companies who continue to abuse our bodies and our environment, then hopefully they'll change their noxious ways. It's all about choice, and in my opinion, going green shouldn't be half-assed. The decision is yours.

For more information on the toxins in our beauty products, check out these great resources: safecosmetics.org, ewg.org (Environmental Working Group) and cosmeticsdatabase.com.

An awesome book on going green on the outside and living an eco-friendly life is *Gorgeously Green* by Sophie Uliano (gorgeouslygreen.com).

· · ·

The Most Common Toxic Chemicals in Your Skin-Care Products

1,4 Dioxane
Alcohol, isopropyl (SD-40)
Ammonium laureth sulfate (ALES)
Ammonium lauryl sulfate (ALS)

Chlorde (stearalkonium, benzalkonium, cetrimonium and
    cetalkonium)
Chloromethylisothiazolinone and isothiazolinone
Cocoamidopropyl betaine (CABP)
Collagen and hydrolyzed collagen

DEA, MEA and TEA
Dimethicone
Disodium (oleamide sulfosuccinate, laureth sulfosuccinate and
    dioctyl sulfosuccinate)
Dioctyl sulfosuccinate
Diazolidinyl urea and DMDM hydantoin

Elastin
Emollients (silicone derived and natural)
FD&C color pigments
Formaldehyde
Fragrance
Glycerin
Hydrolyzed animal protein
Hydroquinone

Imidazolidinyl urea

Lanolin
Lauryl and cocoyl sarcosine

continued

Methicone
Mercury
Mineral oil

Parabens (methyl, propyl, butyl and ethyl)
Paraffin wax/oil
Petroleum products
Polyethylene, polyethylene glycol (PEG) and polyoxyethylene
Propylene/butylenes glycol
Phthalates

Sodium fluoride
Sodium hydroxide
Sodium laureth sulfate (SLES)
Sodium lauryl sulfate (SLS)
Sodium methyl cocoyl taurate
Sodium lauryl sarcosinate
Sodium cocoyl sarcosinate
Stearalkonium chloride

Talc
Toluene

Battling the Branch

$\mathcal{A}$T THIS POINT, you are well on your way to being a healthy and chill chick. Rock on with your bad self! By now, I hope I have pounded into your pretty little head how utterly important it is for you to follow a clean, healthy, organic and nondead diet, get your seven to eight hours of sleep every night, CTFO and get your one-life-to-live body in the best health possible to prevent future diseases.

This chapter is the icing on the new you cake. It's filled with tips for treating your branch health-care issues.

"Branch? Am I a tree now?"

LOL. Let me explain. The natural, simple and sometimes ancient tidbits found throughout this chapter are for ironing out the little healthcare kinks that may be lurking even after you've amply adapted to your new Chill Out and Get Healthy lifestyle. The advice here will help you with treating what we in Chinese Medicine call branch symptoms. These are issues like headaches, yeast infections, heartburn and insomnia. You see, CM views a yeast infection as a result of a backed-up and phlegmy digestive system; a headache is often the result of poor Qi and blood circulation; insomnia can be the result of anxiety. The yeast infection, headache and insomnia are the branches; the phlegmy digestive system, poor circulation and anxiety are the root issues.

"Root?"

Your internal health is the root. Think of yourself as a big ol' maple tree—without strong, deep roots that are flourishing and circulating ample nutrients to the rest of the tree, the branches won't look or feel so great.

Ladies, the information in the rest of this book is for fixing and maintaining your root—this chapter is just to help you manage a nagging branch issue while you're working on the root. YOU have to live the Chill Out and Get Healthy life to rectify your root. YOU must apply all the other tools I've given you throughout this book to get your root in tip-top, nutrient-rich, freaking fabulous health. Because, like I said from the get-go, this is your process. I'm just here to give you advice and help you along the path to optimal health.

Hey, if you're following all the advice found here in this book, and working on your root, you may not even need the tips found in this chapter. But I'm sure they'll come in handy. Even a body in optimal health experiences a kink or two from time to time.

Here's a list of the most common branch issues and the pages where you can find the oh-so-easy-to-do, natural and sometimes ancient solutions for how to deal with them.

• SLEEPING BEAUTY STILL CAN'T SLEEP •

To recap from chapter 2, you should be getting seven to eight hours of sleep every night. You should wake up—most mornings—feeling rested and rejuvenated. You shouldn't have sleep-deprivation dark circles under your eyes, feel like the walking dead or need that Venti latte to wake your ass up.

So, what to do if you really feel like, at this point, you are treating your body in the best possible way and you still can't get a good night's sleep?

- Prepare your sleeping sanctuary. Your bed should be your cozy, comfy "oh I want to sleep (and have sex) there" place. Invest in some satin sheets or find a way to spruce up the place. Learn to love your bed. And remember, your bed should be for sleep and sex, nothing more! FYI: couples who have a TV in their bedroom have less sex than those who don't! For the love of sex, NO TV in bed!
- Lights out. Just like in summer camp. Thirty minutes before bedtime turn off the TV, silence your phone, turn off your BlackBerry and get ready for bed. These electronic devices are way too stimulating and can prevent you from having a good night's sleep.
- CTFO at night. Find a quiet place and take a five-minute CTFO break twenty minutes before you plan on going to bed, noticing where you are holding tension in your body and the thoughts that are still on your mind. Just chill out,

breathe, let the day go and let your body and mind unwind (go back to chapter 3 and review how to CTFO). Here's an idea: do your nighttime CTFO while taking an ooh-la-lavender bath (mentioned below).

- Nighttime journaling. After lights out and your five-minute CTFO break, get into bed, turn on a lamp with soft lighting, get out your journal and write. Take three minutes to just mentally unload. Write about the thoughts that came up during your CTFO break or make yourself a task list for the next day. Allow yourself to let go of the things you can't control at ten p.m. while you're sitting in your bed. It's hard to fall asleep when you have a thousand things on your mind.

- Take a calcium supplement twenty minutes before bedtime. Remember that old wives' tale about a warm glass of milk to help you sleep? Well, that's because calcium is a natural sedative and can really help you fall and stay asleep. If you're not up for drinking the warm milk (or if maybe you're lactose intolerant), take a whole-food, near one hundred percent absorbable calcium supplement. My favorite brands are NutriHarmony, Dr. Ron's and Garden of Life. Take one thousand milligrams per day: five hundred milligrams in the morning and five hundred milligrams twenty minutes before bed.

- Ooh-la-lavender bath. Add four to five drops of lavender essential oil to a tub of hot water and get in. Chill out. Lavender is very soothing and relaxing and the heat from the bath helps stimulate the secretion of melatonin (the brain chemical that helps you sleep).

- Dream makeover. If you suffer from recurring nightmares or disturbing dreams—remodel them. Take time during your day, or at night before bed, and rewrite your dreams the way you wish for them to turn out. Sometimes people have recurring dreams about people who have died. If this is you, write out what you want to say to that person, then reread it before bed and re-create your dreams. In CM we see dreams, especially disturbing ones, as a sign of restless sleep, so ultimately our dreams shouldn't be stirring us up. If you're having dreams that you remember (not everyone remembers their dreams), the goal here is to make them as peaceful as possible.

- Nighttime grind. Do you wake up with a headache, or a sore jaw? Do you notice if you grind your teeth at night? Has your dentist told you that you grind your teeth? According to CM, if you grind your teeth at night or have TMJ (temporomandibular joint pain), you have repressed emotions. Go back to chapter 4 and work out your mental state. Definitely incorporate the nighttime journaling into your daily routine. Night guards work for a lot of people too; talk to your dentist about getting fitted for one. Massaging your masseter (jaw) muscle during the day will help the TMJ. The way you find this muscle is to place your pointer and third finger on the angle of your jawbone and clench your teeth. The muscle that pops up when you clench is your masseter muscle. After you've found the masseter muscle, relax your clenched face, take the tip of your thumb and massage the muscle.

- Restlessness. For those of you who wake up at night and can't get back to sleep, DON'T turn on the TV (remember, your bed is for sleep and sex, that's it!). Get out your journal and write about the things that are stirring in your head, take a CTFO break or have a conversation with yourself. Ask yourself questions like, What's on my mind that I can't sleep? What's up? And just talk it out with yourself. Get over whatever is keeping you stirring. And definitely go back to chapters 3 and 4 and learn to manage your emotions.

- Exercise. Do your best to get in some type of daily exercise. The endorphins (natural brain chemicals in your body) that are released in response to exercise (and orgasms!) have a "feel-good" effect on the body and have been shown to play a large role in our ability to fall asleep faster.

- Have sex. For the same endorphin-release reason that exercise works to calm you and help you fall asleep, sex—orgasmic sex, that is—works too.

- No caffeine after twelve p.m.! That's noon. Bottom line. No exceptions. That includes coffee-flavored ice cream, chocolate, Red Bull and iced tea.
- Avoid spicy foods after lunch. Spicy foods have the same speedlike effect as caffeine and can make you restless before bedtime.

Sleeping Pills

Sure, once in a while during a very stressful time (like a major emotional upheaval or recovery from a trauma), these medications are useful—perhaps vital. But dependency on a pill to sleep through the night isn't healthy.

If you habitually rely on sleep meds—you really need to get to the root of your sleeping issues. Go back to chapters 3 and 4 and work on managing your stress and your head space. And, if you're up for getting needled, find yourself a local acupuncturist at nccaom.org—acupuncture is great for treating insomnia.

· NOT SO SMOOTH ·

Digestion should be easy and smooth with minimal gas and discomfort. If it's not, you really need to tune in to the foods you are eating that your body's having a hard time digesting. If even after following the nutritional advice in chapters 5 and 6—including kicking sugar and soy—you are still having a hard time digesting your foods, I urge you to go one step further and eliminate dairy and wheat from your diet to see if either of them is the culprit (or if both are). Sure, it's not the easiest thing to do, but boy, oh boy, your health is worth it. Check out the "Weigh-in on Wheat" info box in chapter 7 to see if you have symptoms of a wheat intolerance; another great resource you'll want to look at is Glutenfree.com.

- Rub your feet or have someone else do it. Yup, rubbing at the webbing between your second and third toes will help settle your heartburn. This acupressure point is great for relieving heartburn and hiccups.
- Don't eat too fast and don't lie down directly after eating.
- Chew your food *completely*. When oversized food particles wind up in the stomach, the body needs to release extra acid to digest them.
- Avoid spicy foods, fried foods and greasy foods at all costs. In particular, onions, garlic, tomatoes, chocolate, wine, soda, beer and coffee are common heartburn culprits. Don't eat them!
- Are you taking aspirin or ibuprofen (like Advil, Midol or Motrin) a couple of times per week for several weeks at a time? If so, cut back. Both have been shown to increase the incidence of heartburn.
- Manage your stress. Stress can be a major trigger of heartburn. Go back to chapter 3 and really learn to CTFO.
- At the first sign of heartburn, put a hot-water bottle on your tummy and drink warm water. Both will help settle your stomach.
- Eat foods that will absorb the extra stomach acid, like whole-grain crackers, brown rice and oatmeal.
- Take an enteric-coated peppermint-oil supplement. Peppermint aids in healing and digestion, and also relieves upset stomach, gas and bloating. The key here is that it must be taken in enteric-coated capsule form to prevent the oil from being released before it reaches the colon. Do not take any other form of peppermint, as it can exacerbate heartburn. Good brands are Enzymatic Therapy and Natural Factors.
- Drink some chamomile or dandelion-root tea. Alvita teas are my favorite.
- Make some homemade ginger ale: cut yourself a couple slices of fresh gingerroot. Using a spoon, smash the ginger

at the bottom of a glass, add seltzer water and drink (if you need some sweetness, add a touch of agave nectar or stevia).

- Take a probiotic supplement daily. The flora-restoring bacteria found in probiotics promote a healthy digestive tract and will help with your heartburn. My favorite brands are Culturelle and Genestra's HMF Forte. FYI: eating a probiotic-enriched yogurt per day instead won't cut it, as you'd need to eat ten yogurts to get the same amount of healthy bacteria in one capsule of Culturelle. This is one pill I think you should pop!

A Word About Antacids

Yes, antacids like Tums, Pepcid and Nexium effectively block stomach acid, but at the same time, they also prevent the absorption of nutrients and will slow down your digestion. In the long run, these meds will make your indigestion worse, because the stomach acids that they block are imperative to metabolizing the food you eat. Yikes!

Also, many popular antacids carry with them uncomfortable side effects like constipation, diarrhea, gas, bloating and a "rebound effect" (meaning your stomach is now making more acid than it once did).

RAVENOUS HUNGER

- Chances are, if you're too hungry—meaning nothing satisfies your hunger or you're continually ravenous or hungry a half hour after eating—you're not eating enough protein. Protein is optimal for satisfying our hunger because it gives our body the nutrients it needs to function. When we eat protein with every meal, we should be satisfied and not crave more food. Having protein, starting with breakfast and then with every meal thereafter, you should be able to curb an out-of-control appetite.

- Snack on nuts. Nuts are jam-packed with protein. A handful of almonds is great for curbing cravings, especially sugar cravings.
- Go to your doctor and get your thyroid checked. Sometimes excessive hunger is a sign of hyperthyroidism (see info box in chapter 7 for signs and symptoms of hyperthyroidism). And sometimes you may have symptoms of hyperthyroidism, but your blood work doesn't indicate a thyroid disorder. Either way, seeking the advice and treatment of an NCCAOM-certified acupuncturist and herbalist can really help you feel better (go to nccaom.org to find a practitioner in your area).
- Drink water. If you're not drinking enough water, you may feel hungry when you're actually just thirsty. Remember to drink half your body weight in ounces of water daily (unless you have only one kidney, in which case you should drink one-fourth of your weight in ounces of water).

THE BIG BLOAT

If you're feeling bloated and full, there's a good chance your gut is full of food that it can't digest. So focus on cleaning up your diet and eating as clean and nondead as possible. Go back to chapters 5 and 6 and really focus on changing your diet—it'll change your life. As well, try some of the following.

- Add a little spice to your life. Drink hot water with spices like ginger, turmeric, cumin, coriander, chili pepper or red or black pepper (choose one or two from this list and give it a try). All these spices work great for boosting your metabolism and improving digestion.
- Be sure to poop regularly. If you're not taking a solid, ohh-that-felt-good poop on a daily basis, food isn't moving through your system and you will feel bloated and full.
- Take a probiotic supplement daily. The flora-restoring bacteria found in these products promote a healthy digestive

tract and will help keep your colon moving. My favorite brands are Culturelle and Genestra's HMF Forte. Remember: eating a probiotic-enriched yogurt per day instead won't cut it, as you'd need to eat ten yogurts to get the same amount of healthy bacteria as in one capsule of Culturelle. This is one pill I think you should pop!

- Make some homemade ginger ale: cut yourself a couple slices of fresh gingerroot. Using a spoon, smash the ginger at the bottom of a glass, add seltzer water and drink (if you need some sweetness, add a touch of agave nectar or stevia).

- Taking digestive enzymes can help you too. Similase by Tyler is one of my favorite enzymatic products. I don't recommend you take this type of supplement forever, nor on a regular basis, as your body can get too used to it and stop making its own enzymes, but I do recommend it for the occasional I've-had-a-big-meal-and-my-tummy-feels-all-backed-up use. Take no more than once a week. And, if you are on any medications (especially an antacid), speak with your doctor before taking it.

- Go to your doctor and get your thyroid checked. Sometimes a slow metabolism is a sign of hypothyroidism. And sometimes you may have symptoms of hypothyroidism (check out what the symptoms of hypothyroidism are in the info box back in chapter 7), but your blood work doesn't indicate a thyroid disorder. Either way, seeking the advice and treatment of an NCCAOM-certified acupuncturist and herbalist can really help you feel better (go to nccaom.org to find a practitioner in your area).

TOOT, TOOTS

Gas is normal from time to time. But like I said in chapter 2, belching or farting is a clear-cut sign of indigestion. These lovely little bubbles are your body's odorific way of saying "Hey, lady, I can't metabolize this food!" Go back and apply all the information from chapters 5 and 6. Try some of these tips to battle your body's bubbles:

- Add a little spice to your life. Drink hot water with spices like ginger, turmeric, cumin, coriander, chili pepper or red or black pepper (choose one or two of these and give it a try). All these spices work great for boosting your metabolism and improving digestion.
- Drink a mug of dandelion-root or ginger tea after meals. My favorite brand is Alvita teas.
- Chew on some fresh ginger. Cut yourself a small slice of fresh ginger and gnash on it for a few minutes.
- Make some homemade ginger ale: cut yourself a couple slices of fresh gingerroot. Using a spoon, smash the ginger at the bottom of a glass, add seltzer water and drink (if you need some sweetness, add a touch of agave nectar or stevia).
- Take a probiotic supplement daily. The flora-restoring bacteria found in these products promote a healthy, gasless digestive tract. My favorite brands are Culturelle and Genestra's HMF Forte. FYI: eating a probiotic-enriched yogurt per day instead won't cut it; you'd need to eat ten yogurts to get the same amount of healthy bacteria that one capsule of Culturelle gives you. This is one pill I think you should pop!
- Rub your tummy in a clockwise motion (as if you are the clock). For best results, use a little ginger oil.
- Castor oil tummy packs. If you are suffering and feel all gassy and backed up, get yourself some castor oil, but don't drink it! Castor oil is used externally to improve liver function, reduce inflammation and improve digestion. Just take a palmful of castor oil, spread it evenly over a clean lower abdomen (don't spread it on any area where there is an open wound or where the skin is broken), cover the oiled area with a sheet of Saran wrap and then place a heating pad or hot-water bottle over the Saran wrap. Leave on for

ten to twenty minutes. This is oh-so-soothing and will really relieve your discomfort and help you poop! FYI: while you're lying there with the castor oil pack on your tummy, it's a great time to take a CTFO break!

- If all else fails, you may want to see if you have some food intolerances (especially dairy and/or wheat). Eliminate these foods from your diet and see if the gas doesn't go away (and read the "Weigh-in on Wheat" box back in chapter 7 for more information).
- Avoid all dairy products and foods that are greasy, fried and fatty. These foods are notoriously hard to digest and will complicate your digestive matters more!

• POOPING PROBLEMS •

As we talked about in chapter 2, you should be pooping regularly (preferably daily, but at least five days per week); it should be formed in one six-inch-or-so-long banana-shaped piece, leave you feeling completely evacuated and pass out of you smoothly without sweat, grunts or groans. I have to admit, achieving this state of pristine pooping is difficult but by no means unattainable. Following a healthy and clean diet, along with getting ample sleep and paying attention to the way your body reacts to the foods you eat, will get you there. In the meantime, these tips will help you on your path to bowel-movement bliss.

CONSTIPATION

- Drink plenty of water! Remember, half your body weight in ounces of water is a good goal to shoot for daily (one-fourth your body weight if you have one kidney).
- Start your day off with hot water and lemon. Fill a mug with hot water and squeeze the juice from half a lemon into it. Drink it before you eat or drink anything else. For a little

more de-constipating power, add some lemon, orange or ginger zest to the mixture and drink it up. Enjoy.

- Cut your regular meal portions in half, and rather than eating three meals per day, have six smaller meals or snacks throughout the day, and eat them SLOWLY. Taste each bite. Enjoy what you are eating. Be grateful for your food.

- Taking digestive enzymes can help you too. Similase by Tyler is one of my favorite enzymatic products. I don't recommend you take this type of supplement forever, nor on a regular basis, as your body can get too used to it and stop making its own enzymes, but I do recommend it for the occasional I've-had-a-big-meal-and-my-tummy-feels-all-backed-up use. Take no more than once a week. And, if you are on any medications (especially an antacid), speak with your doctor before taking it.

- Castor oil tummy packs. If you are suffering and feel all backed up, get yourself some castor oil, but don't drink it! Castor oil is used externally to improve liver function, reduce inflammation and improve digestion. Just take a palmful of castor oil, spread it evenly over a clean lower abdomen (don't spread it on any area where there is an open wound or where the skin is broken), cover the oiled area with a sheet of Saran wrap and then place a heating pad or hot-water bottle over the Saran wrap. Leave on for ten to twenty minutes. This is oh-so-soothing and will really relieve your discomfort and help you poop! FYI: while you're lying there with the castor oil on your tummy, it's a great time to take a CTFO break!

- Take a probiotic supplement daily. The flora-restoring bacteria found in these products promote a healthy digestive tract and will render you regular. My favorite brands are Culturelle and Genestra's HMF Forte. Eating a probiotic-enriched yogurt per day instead won't cut it; you'd need to eat ten yogurts to get the same amount of healthy bacteria that one capsule of Culturelle gives you.

DIARRHEA

- Eat a cup of cooked whole-grain brown rice. Rice is a natural binder and will help settle your stomach.
- Drink some hot water with fresh ginger and orange or tangerine peel. Get yourself a chunk of fresh gingerroot and grate a teaspoon of it into a mug of hot water; add a couple of small pieces of the rind from either an orange or a tangerine. Drink. Ginger and the rind of oranges and tangerines are all regularly used in CM; they are great for relieving an upset tummy and improving digestion.
- Avoid all dairy products and foods that are greasy and fatty. These foods are hard to digest and will worsen your digestive issues!
- Take a probiotic supplement daily. The flora-restoring bacteria found in these products promote a healthy digestive tract and will render you regular. My favorite brands are Culturelle and Genestra's HMF Forte. FYI: eating a probiotic-enriched yogurt per day instead won't cut it, as you'd need to eat ten yogurts to get the same amount of healthy bacteria that one capsule of Culturelle gives you. This is one pill I think you should pop!

· VAG ISSUES ·

Ladies, a word here before we begin: if you are experiencing any of the below on a regular basis, SEE YOUR GYNO! It's imperative that a possible infection and/or an STD is ruled out and treated if necessary. Any untreated vag issue can lead to more serious issues like infertility and pelvic inflammatory disease. Don't play games with your vagina!

URINARY TRACT INFECTIONS (UTIs)

Word to the wise: these recommendations are for the early stages of a UTI or to prevent recurrent UTIs (if you've never had a UTI, check out the symptoms listed in the box on this page). But remember, if your symptoms are severe, with a high fever and visibly bloody urine, *see your doctor.*

Possible Symptoms of a UTI

- Urinary frequency
- Urinary urgency
- Burning sensation with urination
- Cloudy urine
- Visible blood in urine
- Fever and chills
- Pain or muscle spasms in genital area
- Lower-abdominal pressure
- Back pain

- At the first sign of a UTI—drink loads of water!
- Cranberries, cranberries, cranberries! Cranberry juice has been shown to prevent the development of UTIs by decreasing the ability of the E. coli bacteria to stick to the lining of the urinary tract. You can add to the loads of water you are already drinking with one hundred percent pure, NOT-from-concentrate cranberry juice (good brands are R.W. Knudsen and Mountain Sun). I like to mix one part of one hundred percent pure cranberry juice with two parts water. Try to consume eight to sixteen ounces of the one hundred percent pure juice per day at the onset of UTI symptoms.
- If drinking all that juice seems overwhelming to you, you can take cranberry-extract pills. Taking six hundred to one thousand milligrams of cranberry extract a day will help with your symptoms. Good brands are Pure Encapsulations and Nature's Way.
- Garlic. Garlic has antiviral, antifungal and antibacterial activity and can help ward off a minor infection. If you're daring,

you can eat a clove or two of fresh garlic per day, or make yourself some garlic tea. Put two cloves of garlic in a mug, crush with a spoon, add hot water and drink. You can also take garlic in pill form (make sure it's enteric coated). Best brand: Integrative Therapeutics.

- Pee immediately after sex! No exceptions.
- Take a probiotic supplement daily. The healthy flora-restoring bacteria found in these products help your body fight the bacteria that causes UTIs. My favorite brands are Culturelle and Genestra's HMF Forte. FYI: eating a probiotic-enriched yogurt per day instead won't cut it, as you'd need to eat ten yogurts to get the same amount of healthy bacteria that one capsule of Culturelle gives you. This is one pill I think you should pop!
- Medicinal mushrooms: eat medicinal mushrooms, namely, maitake, shiitake, reishi (aka ganoderma lucidum or ling zhi) and wood ear (aka black mushrooms). These mushrooms are kick-ass immunity-enhancing foods that have been a part of CM healing tradition for centuries. These fantabulous fungi are used to enhance the immune system, fight off cancer and boost postnatal essence.
- If you notice that you are getting recurring UTI symptoms directly after sex, in addition to the no-exception peeing-after-sex rule, get your partner on a probiotic too, because your partner could have a bacterial overgrowth that's causing you to get chronic infections.
- Corn silk. Corn silk (it's actually the yellowish threadlike strands found inside a husk of corn) is an herb used in CM to promote urination and relieve the symptoms of a UTI. Drink three cups of Alvita brand corn silk tea per day or take six capsules per day of Nature's Way corn silk at the first sign of a UTI.
- Sitz it. You can purchase inexpensive sitz baths that fit over the toilet bowl, or you can fill your bathtub about one-fifth of the way with just enough water to cover your lower abdomen.

Basically, you're steeping yourself in herbs that will help you fight this UTI. At the first sign of a UTI, draw a warm bath. To the warm water add four crushed garlic cloves, one cup of Bragg's unpasteurized vinegar and the contents of four Nature's Way corn silk capsules or two Alvita corn silk tea bags. Sit for fifteen minutes. Repeat two to three times per day.

- See an NCCAOM-certified acupuncturist and herbalist for an individualized Chinese herbal formula to help treat your condition (go to nccaom.org to find a practitioner in your area).

YEAST INFECTIONS

According to CM theory, the number one way to treat and prevent yeast infections is by following a clean diet and avoiding all breads (including wheat and rye), dairy products, cheeses of all kinds (including cottage cheese), alcohol and ANY dead, processed food that contains added sugar. You see, all these foods are phlegmy—you remember phlegm from chapter 5, right? Phlegm is NOT our friend, and phlegm in your body feeds the yeast overgrowth that causes a yeast infection. So following the advice in chapter 5 is your best way to prevent a yeast infection.

Here are some additional remedies you can try to help your body be yeast-infection free!

- Garlic. Garlic is an herb used in CM for its antiviral, antifungal and antibacterial activity and can help ward off a minor infection. If you're daring, eat a clove or two of fresh garlic per day. Or make yourself some garlic tea. Put two cloves of garlic in a mug, crush with a spoon, add hot water and drink. You can also take garlic in pill form (be sure it's enteric coated). Best brand: Integrative Therapeutics.
- Drink loads of water. Remember, shoot for half your body weight in ounces of water (or if you have only one kidney, one-fourth your weight). For example, if you weigh 150 pounds, you should be drinking 75 ounces of water per day.

- Vinegar-tampon trick. Because of the acidic nature of vinegar, it is a great topical treatment for the relief of yeast-infection discomfort; vinegar helps restore the normal pH of the vagina and fights off a yeast overgrowth. Here's what you do: into a clean glass, pour approximately one cup of distilled white wine vinegar. Take a new tampon out of its wrapper (keeping it in its applicator—plastic applicators work best) and submerge the tampon in the white wine vinegar until most of the vinegar is soaked up. Then insert the tampon vaginally. I recommend that the first time you do this, you leave the tampon in for only one or two minutes, just to be sure it doesn't further irritate your situation. You can do this tampon trick several times per day, leaving the tampon in for an hour each time.
- Take a probiotic supplement daily. The healthy flora-restoring bacteria found in these products help your body fight the bacterial overgrowth that causes a yeast infection. My favorite brands are Culturelle and Genestra's HMF Forte. FYI: eating a probiotic-enriched yogurt per day instead won't cut it, as you'd need to eat ten yogurts to get the same amount of healthy bacteria that one capsule of Culturelle gives you. This is one pill I think you should pop!
- Apply probiotics directly on your vagina. Yup, buy powdered probiotics and using a clean dry cloth, pat your external vagina with the powder.
- Take apple cider vinegar (enteric-coated) pills to help restore the pH balance in your body and vagina. I don't have a fave brand, just be sure that what you buy is enteric coated.
- If you notice that you are getting recurring yeast infections from sex, get your partner on a probiotic too.
- Medicinal mushrooms: eat medicinal mushrooms, namely, maitake, shiitake, reishi (aka ganoderma lucidum or ling zhi) and wood ear (aka black mushrooms). These mushrooms are kick-ass immunity-enhancing foods that have been a part of CM healing tradition for centuries. These fantabulous

fungi are used to enhance the immune system, fight off cancer and boost postnatal essence.

- Drink two cups of Alvita dandelion-root tea per day. Dandelion root is an herb used extensively in CM, as it has antibacterial properties and will help your body fight off a yeast infection.
- Sitz it. At the first sign of a yeast infection, draw a warm bath, filling the tub about one-fifth of the way, just enough to cover your lower abdomen. To the warm water add four crushed garlic cloves, one cup of Bragg's unpasteurized vinegar and the contents of two Alvita dandelion tea bags. Sit for fifteen minutes. Repeat two to three times per day.

DISCHARGE OVERLOAD

As I said in chapter 2, the only time you should regularly see vaginal discharge is right around ovulation; it should be egg-whitish in color. Anything else is not normal and could signify an underlying infection or an STD. Girl, if you are seeing abnormal vaginal discharge on a regular basis—not just around ovulation—you should see your gyno and rule out an infection or STD.

Excessive vaginal discharge in CM is also a sign of your insides being phlegm filled and turbid. Be sure to follow the dietary advice in chapter 5 to clear up a phlegmy digestive system that may be causing you to have too much vaginal discharge. In addition, using some of the following tips can help you out.

- Take a probiotic supplement daily. The healthy flora-restoring bacteria found in these products help your body fight the bacterial overgrowth that could be causing excessive vaginal discharge. My favorite brands are Culturelle and Genestra's HMF Forte. FYI: eating a probiotic-enriched yogurt per day instead won't cut it, as you'd need to eat ten yogurts to get the same amount of healthy bacteria as one capsule of Culturelle.

- Drink two cups of Alvita dandelion-root tea per day. Dandelion root is used extensively in CM, as it has antibacterial properties and will help your body fight off a vaginal infection (any infection, in fact).
- Medicinal mushrooms: Eat medicinal mushrooms, namely, maitake, shiitake, reishi (aka ganoderma lucidum or ling zhi) and wood ear (aka black mushrooms). These mushrooms are kick-ass immunity-enhancing foods that have been a part of CM healing tradition for centuries. These fantabulous fungi are used to enhance the immune system, fight off cancer and boost postnatal essence.
- Avoid—at all costs—dairy, sugar, white flour and wine. As I said in chapter 5, these foods are phlegm producing and will worsen any excess-phlegmy sticky-discharge-producing situation.
- Vinegar-tampon trick. Because of the acidic nature of vinegar, it is a great topical treatment for excessive vaginal discharge; vinegar helps restore the normal pH of the vagina and fights off a yeast overgrowth. Here's what you do: into a clean glass, pour approximately one cup of distilled white wine vinegar. Take a new tampon out of its wrapper (keeping it in its applicator—plastic applicators are best) and submerge the tampon in the white wine vinegar until most of the vinegar is soaked up. Then insert the tampon vaginally. The first time you do this, leave the tampon in for only a minute or two, just to be sure it doesn't further irritate your situation. If all goes well, you can do this tampon trick several times per day, leaving the tampon in for an hour each time.

VAGINAL DRYNESS

Vaginal dryness is common in menopausal women, but it shouldn't be common in women in their twenties, thirties or forties. Girl, well into your forties, you should be a lusciously lubricated, raging and ravenous horn dog. So what to do if you're dry as a bone?

In CM we see vaginal dryness often in conjunction with dryness elsewhere in the body, and our goal is to nourish this dryness from the inside out and improve blood flow and circulation to the lower abdomen (because if you encourage blood flow in a certain area, tissues in that area will get nourished). We also look into the potential mental and emotional causes of vaginal dryness—either a woman just isn't into the sex (or her partner) or she has emotions surrounding the act of sex that prevent her from becoming wet. From a Western perspective, the most common cause of vaginal dryness is an estrogen deficiency (estrogen, a major female hormone in the body, helps maintain vaginal lubrication, elasticity and health), so it is often treated with the application of estrogen-based creams. Yes, for most women, these estrogen-based creams will help with vaginal dryness, but they are not fixing the root of the problem. To fix the root, you need to balance your hormones (go back to chapter 7 and follow my recommendations), manage your stress levels (go back and reread chapter 3) and maybe even explore your sexual head space (go back to chapter 4 and work it out). In the meantime, try some of these natural recommendations to deal with your dryness from the inside out:

- Evening primrose oil (EPO). Applying EPO inside your vagina—as far up as your cervix—can really help with vaginal dryness, as this oil encourages your body's production of estrogen. Buy EPO in capsule form, pop open two capsules and squeeze the oil out onto clean fingers. Insert your oiled fingers into your vagina—going as high up as you can—and wipe the oil onto the walls of your vagina. What to do if you're not comfy sticking your fingers into your vag? *Get over it!* If you're struggling with uncomfortable, ouch-it-hurts vaginal dryness, this can really help you. Get over it, girl, and give it a shot. Pregnant-gals warning: this is NOT for you, as EPO also has the ability to induce uterine contractions and can send you into early labor. In your case, applying vitamin E oil the same way will work for relieving vaginal dryness.

- Essential fatty acids (EFAs). Taking an EFA supplement can really help out dryness in ANY area of the body, as these fats help your body produce optimal levels of hormones and stay hydrated and lubricated. As I said in chapter 6, my favorite form of EFAs is in either fish oil or cod-liver oil. Two of the brands I recommend are Green Pasture's (greenpasture.org) and Nordic Naturals.

- Drink loads of water. Any dryness symptom can be a sign of dehydration. Remember, half your body weight in ounces of water is what's recommended.

- Vitamin E oil, cocoa butter or emu oil. With clean hands massage any one of these natural lubricators on the inside walls of your vagina, just as I recommended with the EPO. Be sure these products are all-natural, chemical free and one hundred percent pure.

- Do some introspection and ask yourself, Am I into my partner? Sometimes you have vaginal dryness because you're just not that into the partner you're with. Ask yourself if this is the case. If it is—make a change in your relationship. The tools in chapter 4, especially in the "Acknowledge Your Desires" section, are great for helping you figure out what you need from your life.

- Is something else on your mind? Ask yourself and find out. Go back to chapter 3 and learn how to manage your stress so that it doesn't interfere in your intimate life. As I've said on numerous occasions throughout this book, stress causes hormonal imbalances (via the brain chemicals adrenaline and cortisol that stress produces) and this stress-induced hormonal imbalance could be what's making you dry. Darlin', chill out and manage your stress so you can enjoy sex!

CERVICITIS, VAGINITIS AND VAGINOSIS

If you are experiencing symptoms of any of these diseases (see box), you MUST see your gyno to rule out an infection or an STD.

Vag Issues You NEED to See Your Gyno About

Vaginitis: a thick, white, cottage-cheese-ish, odorless discharge with itching and burning of the vagina that is exacerbated by urination or sex.

Vaginosis: a grayish discharge that has a fishlike odor that is present after sex or during your period.

Trichomoniasis: a yellow green "frothy" discharge that may or may not cause itchiness or burning.

Cervicitis: abnormal vaginal bleeding (especially after sex), abnormal vaginal discharge, pain with urination and sex.

In addition, try some of the following tips to help your body and your vag feel better.

- Do some introspection and ask yourself, Am I into my partner? Do I trust my partner? Sometimes our bodies have a pseudo-allergic I'm-just-not-that-into-you reaction to people. And that may just be the case with you. If you are experiencing recurring vag issues, I urge you to look into your relationship and decide if it's what you want, if it's making you happy, if it's making you sick. Use the tools in chapter 4 to get to the root of your emotional desires and needs.
- Are you lubricated enough? Friction, NOT the good kind, can cause vaginal irritation and discomfort, sometimes even bleeding. Try using some of the tips in the "Vaginal Dryness" section to help keep yourself lusciously lubricated.
- Take a probiotic supplement daily. The healthy flora-restoring bacteria found in these products help your body fight the bacterial overgrowth that could be causing excessive vaginal discharge and infection. My favorite brands are Culturelle and Genestra's HMF Forte.
- Medicinal mushrooms: Eat medicinal mushrooms, namely, maitake, shiitake, reishi (aka ganoderma lucidum or ling zhi)

and wood ear (aka black mushrooms). These mushrooms are kick-ass immunity-enhancing (not to mention antiaging and essence-generating) foods that have been a part of CM healing tradition since AD 200. These fantabulous fungi are used to enhance the immune system, fight off cancer and boost postnatal essence.

- Drink two cups of Alvita dandelion-root tea per day. Dandelion root is used extensively in CM, as it has antibacterial properties and will help your body fight off a vaginal infection (any infection to boot).

- Sitz it. At the first sight of abnormal discharge, draw a warm sitz bath, meaning you fill the tub about one-fifth of the way, just enough to cover your butt and your vag. To the warm water add four crushed garlic cloves, one cup of Bragg's unpasteurized vinegar and the contents of two Alvita dandelion tea bags.

- Garlic. Garlic has antiviral, antifungal and antibacterial activity and can help ward off a minor infection. If you're daring, you can eat a clove or two of fresh garlic per day, or make yourself some garlic tea. Put two cloves of garlic in a mug, crush them with a spoon, add hot water and drink. You can also take garlic in pill form—make sure it's enteric coated. Best brand: Integrative Therapeutics.

- Avoid—at all costs—dairy, sugar, white flour and wine. As I said in chapter 5, these foods are phlegm producing and will worsen any excess-phlegmy sticky-discharge-producing situation.

· OUCH, IT HURTS! ·

You should never have pain with intercourse. Sure, right before your period, when your uterus is full of blood, sex can be a little uncomfortable. And if he's *that* well-endowed, it can hurt a bit. But otherwise, sex shouldn't be painful. Pain (like the sharp stabbing kind, or the ouch-it's-irritating kind, or the it's-uncomfortable-and-makes-me-want-to-vomit kind) during sex can be an indication of gynecological problems, such as endometriosis (see box below), pelvic inflammatory disease and vulvodynia (see box on pages 231–32). If you experience pain with sex regularly, *I urge you to see your gyno* and request a transvaginal sonogram to rule out some of these concerns (your doctor may have to do additional tests to rule them all out).

Endometriosis

In the clinic, I see patients who have been diagnosed with endometriosis quite a bit, as it's very often a cause of infertility (I also see a lot of women who haven't been officially diagnosed with endometriosis but do show symptoms of it).

Endometriosis occurs when the tissue—called endometrial tissue—that normally grows inside your uterus grows outside your uterus. This tissue can grow in the ovaries, fallopian tubes, colon, rectum and vagina. The most common symptom of endometriosis is intense pelvic pain. A lot of women I see experience the most pain at ovulation and premenstrually (and some women with endometriosis don't have any pain at all). I find that endometriosis symptoms respond very well to a combined approach of acupuncture, Chinese herbs and strict dietary changes. Removing wheat

continued

and dairy completely from the diet significantly improves endometriosis symptoms.

Keep in mind, a laparoscopy (a minimally invasive surgery where a small incision is made near the belly button to view structures within the abdomen and pelvis) and/or getting a pelvic MRI are the only two ways to definitively diagnose endometriosis.

See a reproductive endocrinologist if you suspect you have endometriosis.

Below are some pointers that can help you feel better regardless of the nature of your vaginal pain:

- Acupuncture. Seeing an acupuncturist who specializes in gynecological issues and disorders of the pelvis can offer you a great amount of relief. Sometimes the pain women experience during sex is due to poor circulation in the lower abdominal area or it could be that the muscles of her pelvic floor are too tight and tense. Seeing a practitioner who is knowledgeable about the female reproductive system and its anatomy and is comfortable with needling muscles of the pelvic floor is imperative. Get a referral to a few local NCCAOM-certified acupuncturists and ask if they have experience in treating your condition (or go to nccaom.org).
- Physical therapy (PT). For the same reason that acupuncture can be helpful, PT can be very useful in treating muscular tension in the pelvic muscles. To find a physical therapist who knows how to help pelvic-floor muscles, check out the following Web sites: National Vulvodynia Association (nva.org) and International Pelvic Pain Society (pelvicpain.org).
- Mayan abdominal massage. This massage technique is very gentle and noninvasive. It works to reposition internal organs that may have shifted (due to diseases such as endometriosis) and increases blood flow, lymph circulation

and Qi flow in the abdominal cavity. Go to www.arvigo-massage.com for more information.

- Positions. Maybe your anatomy is a bit restricted "down there." If you're experiencing pain in only certain positions, don't do them.
- Are you lubricated enough? Friction can cause vaginal irritation and discomfort, sometimes even bleeding. Try using some of the tips in the "Vaginal Dryness" section to help keep yourself lusciously lubricated.
- Avoid—at all costs—dairy, sugar, white flour and wine. These foods are phlegm producing and make any inflammation or pain in your body worse.
- Following a clean and organic diet is key to helping your body recover from diseases like pelvic inflammatory disorder, endometriosis and vulvodynia.
- Do some introspection and ask yourself, Am I into my partner? Do I trust my partner? Sometimes our bodies have a pseudo-allergic I'm-just-not-that-into-you reaction to people. And that may just be the case with you. If you are experiencing recurring vag issues, I urge you to look into your relationship and decide if it's what you want, if it's making you happy, if it's making you sick. Use the tools in chapter 4 to get to the root of your emotional desires and needs.

Didn't Charlotte on SATC Have Vulvodynia?

Yes, she was diagnosed with vulvodynia on *Sex and the City* but unfortunately the severity of the disease was downplayed quite a bit.

Vulvodynia isn't fun. Most women who have it are in so much pain that they can't even use tampons and they definitely can't have sex. Vulvodynia is characterized by chronic pain, burning, stinging and a feeling of rawness, irritation or discomfort of the vulva (aka the vaginal lips). It's not known what causes vulvodynia, but

continued

it usually occurs after an injury or irritation to the nerves that feed into the vaginal lips, from muscular tension in the pelvic region or in response to a candida hypersensitivity (candida is the stuff that causes yeast infections).

Most women with vulvodynia are treated with a host of medications, nerve blocks and sometimes Botox injections into their vaginal lips. Ouch! In my practice, I see that women respond to a multifaceted approach of PT, acupuncture and dietary changes (including a strictly yeast-free diet). Go to NVA.org for more information on vulvodynia.

• I'M SO NOT IN THE MOOD •

As I said in chapter 2 (and earlier in this chapter), in our twenties, thirties and forties we should be raging, ravenous and ready-to-procreate sex goddesses. Period. If you're not, try some of the tips here to lift your lustiness.

- Do some introspection and ask yourself, Am I into my partner? Do I trust my partner? If you have zero lust in your libido, I urge you to look into your relationship and decide if it's what you want, if it's making you happy, if it's making you sick. Use the tools in chapter 4 to get to the root of your emotional desires and needs.
- Is something else on your mind? Ask yourself and find out. Go back to chapter 3 and learn how to manage your stress so that it doesn't interfere in your intimate life. As I've said on numerous occasions throughout this book, stress causes hormonal imbalances (via the brain chemicals adrenaline and cortisol that stress produces) and this stress-induced hormonal imbalance could be what's making your sex drive suck. Chill out and manage your stress so you can get into sex!
- Cordyceps. This is a widely used Chinese herb (it's actually

a fungus) that boosts the immune system, promotes vitality, reduces the signs of aging and enhances libido. New Chapter makes a great organic cordyceps product.

- Out-of-whack hormones. A low sex drive can be an indication of a hormonal imbalance—follow the hormone-balancing diet in chapter 7 to get your body back into hormonal bliss.

- Take cod-liver oil or fish oil. The essential fatty acids that these oils contain play an important role in helping our body produce and regulate hormones. Go back to chapter 6 and reread what I said about them. Two of my favorite brands: Green Pasture's (greenpasture.org) and Nordic Naturals. Take two capsules per day.

- Balance out the Pill. If you're currently taking an oral contraceptive, chances are you have zero sex drive. The Pill shuts down hormonal production in your body to prevent ovulation from occurring. The same hormones that help you ovulate put the lust in your libido. If this sounds like your problem, follow the hormone-balancing recommendations found in chapter 7 and incorporate some of the other advice found here to sexy up your sex drive.

- Mood-altering meds. Pharmaceuticals like antidepressants and antianxiety medications dull your feelings so that you are less sensitive to outside stimuli. By the same token, they'll dull your desire to have sex. If this sounds like what's affecting you, talk with your prescribing doctor about switching to a medication with less libido-reducing power (or talk about whether you really need these meds—maybe you're ready to get off them?).

- Smoking too much pot can seriously suck the lust for sex right out of you (not to mention your lust for life too). You may need to drop the drugs to get your sex life back! Reread chapters 3 and 4 and learn how to handle your emotions.

- Confidence. Girl, have you lost your mojo? Maybe you're not feeling as hot and appealing as you once did? Go back to chapters 4 and 8 and work on boosting your inner beauty. Get your confidence back!

- Use it or lose it. Like I said in chapter 3, sometimes you gotta fake it till you make it. Go back to chapter 4, incorporate the advice I laid down and get back in bed with your partner and rekindle that lovers' lust.

• TOO HOT, TOO COLD •

Too hot? Too cold? Just right? Poor Goldilocks. Fluctuating body temperatures can drive any woman berserk! In CM, we often see temperature fluctuations as a sign of insufficient Qi and blood and/or poor Qi and blood flow. Your insides are overheated or too cold and you need to be brought back into balance. Try some of these recommendations for regulating your body (for more specific advice for you, see an NCCAOM-board-certified acupuncturist and herbalist; go to nccaom.org to find someone in your area).

EXCESSIVE SWEATING

CM is often very successful in treating excessive sweating. Western medicine calls excessive sweating hyperhidrosis, and typically treats it using surgery, medication or Botox injections. CM can treat excessive sweating using acupuncture, Chinese herbs and lifestyle changes. See a local NCCAOM-certified acupuncturist and herbalist for treatment (nccaom.org). Also, be sure to

- Drink plenty of water! With excessive sweating, your body is losing A LOT of precious fluids—replenish them.
- Ask yourself, is anxiety making me sweat? If there's even a smidgen of a chance you think so, go back to chapter 4 and get to the root of it!
- Try eating cooling foods like cucumbers, asparagus, mushrooms, spinach, Swiss chard, watercress, seaweed, kelp,

lemon, watermelons, persimmons, pears and grapefruit. These foods will cool down your overheated insides and can help stop your sweating.

- Eliminate caffeine and spicy foods, as they are very stimulating and can exacerbate excessive sweating.

NIGHT SWEATS

Remember Amanda from chapter 3? She suffered from terrible night sweats. Based on her clinical presentation, I determined that her night sweats were a result of her body becoming overheated and dehydrated because of her repressed emotions and chronic stress. To get to the bottom of your night sweating, make an appointment with your local NCCAOM acupuncturist and herbalist. In the meantime, try some of these tips as well:

- Often, night sweats are indicative of an out-of-whack hormonal system. Go back to chapter 7 and incorporate the hormone-balancing foods into your already clean, organic and nondead diet.
- Stay hydrated! Drink sixteen ounces of cold water before going to bed (not in addition to the "half your weight in ounces of water" rule, though).
- Dress light. Wear loose, comfy and breathable pj's to help maintain your body's temperature at night.
- Take cod-liver oil or fish oil. The essential fatty acids that these oils contain play an important role in helping our body produce and regulate hormones. Go back to chapter 6 and reread what I said about them. Best brands: Green Pasture's and Nordic Naturals.
- Antidepressant medications can often cause night sweats—so if you're on an antidepressant and experiencing night sweats, think back and try to remember if you had night sweats before you began taking your medication. Talk with your prescribing doctor to see if you can switch to

a medication that has fewer side effects (or talk about whether you really need these meds).

TOO COLD

Many women complain they're too cold. In CM theory, we believe that's due to the fact that a lot of women are deficient in blood. Huh? You see, every woman in her reproductive years menstruates (or at least she should) and through menstruation she gives up blood on a monthly basis. This can render a lot of women blood deficient. No, you won't necessarily have anemia according to Western medical-lab tests, but you may show signs of blood deficiency (like being too cold, thin or pale; having low energy, dry skin, dry hair or brittle nails; seeing floaters or spots in your eyes or often having very light periods). CM treatment for being too cold is to nourish and build blood as well as circulate it.

For specific recommendations for you, go to an NCCAOM-certified acupuncturist and herbalist (find one in your area at nccaom.org). In the meantime:

- Try eating more blood-building foods like red meat, beets, green veggies, black cherries, eggs, oysters, almonds, dates and goji berries.
- Drink some turmeric and ginger tea. Turmeric is a CM herb used for improving blood flow and circulation; ginger is a CM herb used for warming up your insides. Combine the two and you have a great circulating and warming tea to enjoy.
- Incorporate warming spices and herbs into your diet like cinnamon, fennel seed, mustard seeds, ginger, pepper (any), basil, clove, coriander, nutmeg, star anise, caraway and rosemary. Cook with them, sprinkle them on your food or make a tea with them.
- Exercise. As I said in chapter 7, everyone's exercise capacities differ. So listen to your body. But the bottom line is, move-

ment will encourage blood flow and circulation and make your body warmer overall. Exercise is especially good for those who suffer from cold hands and feet.

· MY ACHING HEAD ·

Head hurts? Well, it shouldn't. There's a host of reasons for headaches. It's really up to you to consider the foods you eat, the tension in your neck and shoulders, the boulder strapped to your shoulder that's called a handbag, your hormones, any seasonal allergies, whether you grind your teeth at night, or the emotions you may be suppressing, and how one or all of these can be causing your headaches. While you're working on the root problem causing your headaches, here are some branch treatments you can try to give yourself some much-needed relief.

HEADACHES

- **Aspartame.** Avoid aspartame at all costs. Researchers from the University of Washington found a direct correlation between headaches and aspartame intake.
- **Wheat.** Try going without wheat and see if your daily headache doesn't disappear. Often people have a sensitivity to wheat that manifests itself with an oh-so-annoying headache (read more on potential wheat sensitivity in the "Weigh-in on Wheat" info box in chapter 7).
- **The grind.** Grinding your teeth at night or clenching your teeth during your stressful day can cause pretty bad tension headaches. It can also cause TMJ—temporomandibular joint pain. See your dentist and ask if you have signs of TMJ.
- **Stop, drop and sigh.** I recommended this exercise back in chapter 4; you can do it for tension headaches too! To recap, this is what you do: put a Post-it note on a mirror in your bedroom or your computer screen at work or set a daily reminder on your phone that says "SDS." And when you are

reminded, stop what you're doing, drop your tensed-up shoulders (remembering to relax your jaw if you hold tension there too) and let out a long and liberating sigh. AHH-HHHH! In CM theory sighing is the sound of the liver, so it is said that when you let out a deep sigh, you are moving stuck liver Qi and therefore helping your liver detox. This is a nice time-out and is great to do when you are feeling particularly stressed. Sigh your stress and tension away.

- **HORMONES.** Headaches are very often related to a woman's menstrual cycle. Try incorporating the hormone-balancing foods highlighted in chapter 7 into your already clean, organic, nondead and aspartame-free diet and see if that doesn't help your headaches.

- **CTFO.** Headaches can be a side effect of our stressful lives. Remember to take your daily CTFO break. Also, go back to chapter 3 and manage that stress!

- **OOH-LA-LAVENDER.** Get yourself a lavender eye pillow and when you feel a headache coming on, lie down, CTFO and let the lavender relax your headache away. Or try taking a hot bath with four or five drops of lavender essential oil in it. Ooh-la-lavender away your headache.

- **ALL STUFFED UP.** If you notice that your headaches have a stuffed-up-sinusy connection, get yourself a neti pot and use it every single day. This is a nasal irrigation system that will clear your sinuses and leave you breathing like a champ; it helps fight colds too. The first time you use your neti pot, you're going to think I'm crazy, as it can be uncomfortable. But if backed-up or dry sinuses are exacerbating your headaches, you'll thank me.

- **PROLACTIN.** If you've tried everything else and you are still getting bad headaches AND your menstrual cycle is irregular, make an appointment with an endocrinologist and get your prolactin levels checked. Prolactin is a hormone released from the pituitary gland (which is a small gland that sits at the base of your brain). Prolactin is primarily released to promote lactation when a woman is pregnant. Sometimes the pituitary gland grows a benign (noncancerous) tumor that overproduces prolactin and can cause headaches, abnormal menstruation and infertility.

HANGOVERS

Let's face it: we all overindulge from time to time. When you do, try the following to make yourself feel better:

- Eat parsley. Fresh parsley is an herb used in CM specifically for its aromatic properties—its strong flavor and smell—which are said to "open up orifices" like your head that is blocked up and headachy from last night's overindulgence. This aromatic property will also help your nausea and upset stomach.
- Drink lots of water. All day long. Alcohol is überdehydrating.
- Drink hot water with the juice from half a lemon. This is very detoxifying to the liver and will help your body process out all the excess alcohol.
- Eat whole-grain breads or crackers. The fiber in these products will help absorb the excess alcohol in your system and get you on the road to recovery.
- Chew on the rind of an orange, a lemon or a tangerine. These rinds stimulate the digestive system and will help your body digest and process the excess alcohol circulating in your body.
- Don't eat heavy, greasy, fried foods even if you want to. These foods are very hard to digest and will take away energy from your body as it's trying to process out the alcohol. Go for clean, lean and nondead foods.
- Make yourself some barley water and drink it. Simmer one-half cup of pearled barley in one quart of water for twenty minutes. If the barley water becomes too thick to drink comfortably, add more water. Remove from the stove and sieve off the water (the grain can be saved for a soup or a

salad). Add the juice from two lemons to your homemade barley water. Drink five cups throughout the day of your hangover. Barley water is very cleansing to the body and will help cleanse your liver of the excess alcohol. Don't do this if you're gluten sensitive.

· THE LITTLE ENGINE THAT COULDN'T ·

Ladies, you should have enough energy to get through your day. Period. If you don't, even after you've been living the Chill Out and Get Healthy life, try some of these energy-enhancing tips:

- **PROTEIN, PROTEIN, PROTEIN.** Protein gives us *sustainable* energy. Not sugar. Not caffeine. These guys give you a false sense of energy that actually leaves you lower than when you started. Don't use them to boost your energy. Instead, make sure you are eating a clean, organic and protein-rich diet. Make sure you are eating a protein-rich breakfast. And, ladies, remember, you are what you eat—if you eat DEAD, energyless foods, you are going to feel DEAD and energyless.
- **DRINK WATER, NOT RED BULL!** Yes, water will give you energy. It is very cleansing to your body and will promote healthy circulation and drainage that will improve your energy. Remember to drink half your body weight in ounces of water (or one-fourth if you have only one kidney).
- **REGULAR EXERCISE GIVES YOU ENERGY.** Get your butt to the gym. I know when you're tired, the last thing you feel like doing is working out, but you should. The chemicals released by your body during exercise will boost your energy. In fact, a review of scientific studies on exercise and energy published in *Psychological Bulletin* concluded that sedentary people who adopted a regular exercise regimen had more energy than those who didn't. Just do it!
- **CORDYCEPS.** This is a widely used Chinese herb (it's actually

a fungus) that boosts the immune system, promotes vitality, reduces the signs of aging and enhances libido. New Chapter makes a great organic cordyceps product.

- **ASTRAGALUS.** It's a widely used herb in CM for boosting Qi and therefore enhancing one's energy or life force. It also strengthens your immune system. Drink a cup or two of astragalus tea each day. Alvita makes a top-quality astragalus tea.
- **BOREDOM.** Maybe your energy levels are zilch because you're bored? Change your routine. Walk to work. Go to bed early. Take up a new hobby. Go back to chapter 4 and seriously start prioritizing your happiness!
- **DEPRESSION.** Lethargy can definitely be a sign of depression. Go back to chapter 4 and mentally detox. Consider talking to a therapist or a life coach.

· BEING SICK SUCKS ·

As I said, being sick sucks. Heading a cold off at the get-go is absolutely ideal and can cut down on your sniffly, sneezy, can't-get-out-of-bed time. At the first sign of a cold, try these remedies:

- I ♥ Neti Pot. Nasal irrigation has been used for centuries; it removes mucus, pollen and other inhaled debris from your sinuses, soothes the lining of the nose and improves its function. You can use a neti pot daily to improve nasal function, but definitely do it at the first sign of a cold, as excess, thick mucus that lingers in the sinuses is fertile ground for infections and bacteria. Yuck. Nasal irrigation is the only way that thick mucus can be washed out of the nose and it's great for kicking a sinus infection. Do it!
- Garlic. Garlic has antiviral, antifungal and antibacterial activity and can help ward off a minor infection. Try eating a clove or two of fresh garlic per day or make yourself some garlic tea. Put two cloves of garlic in a mug, crush with a

spoon, add hot water and drink. You can also take garlic in pill form—make sure it's enteric coated. Best brand: Integrative Therapeutics.

- Avoid—at all costs—dairy, sugar, white flour and wine. As discussed in chapter 5, these are all extremely phlegmy substances and will feed your cold!
- Drink water! Stay hydrated and wash your cold away.
- Take two thousand milligrams of vitamin C three times per day. Cut back on the vitamin C if you notice you are getting loose stools.
- Steam your cold away. At the first sign of a cold, steam your face. Boil some water, add a few drops of eucalyptus essential oil, throw a towel over your head and steam your face over the mixture (be sure to remove the boiling water from the heat once it's boiled).
- Gargle with salt water. If you have a sore throat, this works like a charm. Do it.
- Honey. If you have a sore throat, drink hot water with a teaspoon of honey. This will really soothe your aching throat.
- Drink hot water with the juice from half a lemon and three slices of fresh ginger at the first sign of a cold. Take this remedy at least three times per day for the first two days you feel symptomatic. It will help detoxify your body of any evil lurking, sickness-causing bacteria. If you have a sore throat, add a teaspoon of honey to this concoction.
- If you have a fever, add to a cup of boiling water two chopped garlic cloves, four slices of fresh ginger, half a chopped onion and a dash of cinnamon and clove. Drink up and get under the covers. This remedy will cause you to sweat out your fever.
- Rest!!! Listen to your body and get yourself better!
- Take a probiotic supplement daily. The healthy flora-restoring bacteria found in these products boost your immune system and help your body fight the bacterial overgrowth that could be causing your cold. My favorite brands are Cul-

turelle and Genestra's HMF Forte. FYI: eating a probiotic-enriched yogurt per day instead won't cut it, as you'd need to eat ten yogurts to get the same amount of healthy bacteria that one capsule of Culturelle gives you. This is one pill I think you should pop!

- Get acupuncture. Acupuncture is great for boosting your immune system and treating colds. Find an NCCAOM-certified acupuncturist in your area at nccaom.org.

All right, ladies, now you have all the Chill Out and Get Healthy quick fixes for the common everyday issues that may ail you. Go out and stock up on fresh gingerroot, garlic, dandelion and corn silk tea, lavender and eucalyptus essential oils, a neti pot and medicinal mushrooms, and be prepared to battle the branch.

But remember one thing: the remedies mentioned in this chapter are just Band-Aid treatments. Yes, they are all-natural Band-Aids, but that doesn't make them all-encompassing. They are still just branch treatments and they do NOT address the underlying issue that is ailing you. The nagging nonsensical quandaries that you deal with on a regular basis are a direct manifestation of a deeper-lying root problem.

Honey, Rome wasn't built in a day and neither was your health (or lack thereof). To fix the root of your health, you gotta live the Chill Out and Get Healthy life. This book has a butt-load of tools to help you do just that. Do yourself the biggest, best favor and use them. Work out the kinks in your body. Renovate your root. Boost your health from the inside out. Girl, get to the root of your problems and get a grip on your health!

Now I'm going to help you bring it on home!

Bringin' it Home

*Y*OU MADE IT to the last chapter! You now have all my best tools, tricks, tips, ideas and tried and tested Chinese Medicine–based, woman-to-woman, emotionally liberating, nutritionally balanced advice that will help you lead the best Chill Out and Get Healthy life ever.

Brava!

Now I'm going to help you bring it home. By that, I mean I'm going to tell you how the Chill Out and Get Healthy life is completely, totally, positively realistic and doable.

Repeat after me:

Everything in Moderation.

Seems simple, right? And it is. Really and truly.

As I've said throughout this book, girl, Be Mod, because life is too freakin' short.

Remember, Being Mod means that eighty to eighty-five percent of the time (five to six days per week) you live a Chill Out and Get Healthy life.

It means that when you're out for dinner on Saturday night and you order dessert, the Chill Out and Get Healthy police aren't going to take you away and hang you by your toes while onlookers throw goji berries at you.

It means that if you miss your CTFO time one day, you're not going to wake up with more wrinkles and gray hair.

It means that if you have one day where you say "f**k it" to your new clean, organic, nondead way of eating, and really fall off the wagon (say with a Mickey D's dollar-menu cheeseburger and fries), tomorrow's a brand-new day for you to get back on the Chill Out and Get Healthy train.

It means that if once in a while your anxiety about the job, the love life and the parents gets a tight hold of you and you need some Xanax (from the prescription that you filled six months ago and rarely take anymore), that's OK because tomorrow is another day and you're in control of life, more than ever before.

It means that if you get a little constipated one week, chances are you're not going to die of colon cancer.

It means that if you use a nongreen beauty product once in a while, the ozone will not crumble, nor will your face.

It means that if you are stressed-out and can't sleep one night during the month, you are not going to wind up infertile.

It means that if you're getting stressed-out that you're not chilling the f**k out, chill, baby! Be Mod. Everything in moderation.

OK, let's break down what you just learned about living your new Chill Out and Get Healthy life.

You learned that I was once like you. I was struggling to be healthy, I was out of touch with how my emotions were weighing me down, stress ruled me and my bowel movements were an explosive, urgent mess! I learned, just as you learned through reading this book, that optimal health and all the perks that come with it (like great skin, a fab fertility quotient, fewer wrinkles, better sleep, regular and oh-so-complete bowel movements and emotional balance) can be achieved by living the Chill Out and Get Healthy life eighty to eighty-five percent of the time. I leaped into the Chill Out and Get Healthy life and you can too!

You learned all about what your health should and should not look like. That it should be like that gorgeous Marc Jacobs bag featured in In Style last month: durable, dependable, functional, always looking and feeling oh-so-fabulous and envied by all. Not that secondhand, ink-stained, battered, I'll-use-it-to-carry-groceries sack you found at the downtown Salvation Army.

You learned that you need to sleep. That you should be getting a good, solid, restful, relaxed and rejuvenating seven to eight hours of sleep each night. You also learned that if you don't get a good night's sleep regularly, you increase your chances of having diabetes, high blood pressure, heart disease and a stroke. Get to sleep, already!

You were reminded that you should be drinking half your body weight in ounces of water each day (for example, 70 ounces of water if you weigh 140 pounds). You learned that drinking room-temperature or hot water, rather than cold water, is best for your digestion and metabolism (unless, of course, you're a Fire Girl). You learned that stuff like Vitaminwater, Gatorade, coffee, Crystal Light and Diet Coke do NOT count as water. Drink the water (not the Kool-Aid), baby!

You were liberated when I told you that you should be hungry in the morning and that you should eat a protein-packed breakfast because it boosts your energy and helps keep your fat-burning metabolism in check. You learned that you should never, ever ignore your hunger, because starvation ruins your metabolism and will cause you to gain weight in the long run. Eat, it does a body good!

You gawked when I told you that digestion should be easy, comfortable and free of any toots or heartburn and that you should not be so bloated after a meal that you have to unbutton your jeans. You said, "Sign me up" when you learned that eating the Chill Out and Get Healthy way will leave you feeling succulently satisfied, nourished and energized. You now know that you should enjoy your food, be grateful for it and eat it slowly—tasting each bite. You now know that having one beautiful, brown, banana-shaped bowel movement that leaves you feeling elatedly oh-so-empty each day represents a strapping immune system. You were reminded that taking laxatives or getting colonics on a regular basis is moronic. Divine Digestion, here you come!

You learned that eating clean, nondead, non-GM and organic food flat-out rocks, boosts your postnatal essence, improves your fertility quotient and keeps the aging demons at bay. Your jaw dropped and you swore off added sugars, soy and white flour forever when you learned that they cause diseases that you don't want. You learned that you should have no more than one serving of organic, hormone-free, antibiotic-free, nonhomogenized, steroid-free, full-fat and grass-fed dairy per day (remember: yogurt excluded). You were given information so that you could figure out if you might be lactose or wheat intolerant. You learned how to properly prepare your foods and how to make some killer hummus. Girl, get down with that nondead way of life.

You were so excited when you learned how to make your precious palace pristine and baby-licious. You learned all about what your period should look like, what ovulation is, when it should occur and what it should look like. You were over the moon when you heard that living the Chill Out and Get Healthy life means having NO PMS. You learned how to manage and prevent annoying vag issues. You now have tools to improve your fertility quotient and create the best damn postnatal essence. Rock on with your bad self!

You learned how to Chill the F**k Out. You were reminded that stress is evil, that it will age the bajeezus out of you and eat up all your precious essence. You learned how to manage your stressors, how to make happiness a priority in your life and that your CTFO time each and every day is key to optimal health. CTFO for life!

You learned how to B.E. C.A.L.M. You were inspired to acknowledge your desires and to wholeheartedly go after them. You were reminded that you love yourself. You now know that saying "I love you" to yourself each and every day is key to optimal health. You learned how to feel your feelings—good and bad—each and every day. You learned how to make your life happen. Girlfriend, you are freaking fabulous!

You learned how to be beautiful from the inside out—and a couple of cool ancient beauty secrets to boot. You now know what the best antiaging foods are, and you're going to eat them. You learned that inner confidence is the foundation of external beauty. And that everlasting beauty doesn't come in a one-hundred-dollar eye cream. Honey, you're hot!

You got the lowdown on nutritional supplements and beauty products. In fact, you're on your way out to buy some cod-liver oil (or fish oil, depending on your needs) right now. You got some great pointers on getting over headaches, tummyaches, insomnia, diarrhea, heartburn, hangovers, yeast infections and cold feet (the physical and mental kind!).

Most important, I hope you learned that the key to succeeding at the Chill Out and Get Healthy life is to try your damnedest to treat your body like it's the most precious place on earth. Sanctify it. Nourish it. Respect it. Love it. Beautify it from the inside out. Keep it clean, organic and green. Fulfill its desires. Work like hell to get rid of the demons. Appreciate its imperfections. And, by all means, run around naked in it while you belt out your favorite mantra.

All right, darlin', you're finally ready to put down this book. First, I want you to affix your everything-in-moderation cap to your pretty little head, take a few deep, I-love-myself-and-I'm-grateful-for-my-life breaths and get ready to take a very confident, my-body-is-the-most-precious-place-on-earth first step into your new-you Chill Out and Get Healthy life! Honey, go out there and make me proud! You can do it. I have faith in YOU!